HEARING EQUALS BEHAVIOR

HEARING EQUALS BEHAVIOR

Guy Bérard, M.D.

Preface by Bernard Rimland, Ph.D.

Afterword by Annabel Stehli

Keats Publishing, Inc. New Canaan, Connecticut

HEARING EQUALS BEHAVIOR is not intended as medical advice. Its intent is solely informational and educational. Please consult a health professional should the need for one be indicated.

Hearing Equals Behavior

Copyright © 1993 by Guy Bérard

Library of Congress Cataloging-in-Publication Data

Bérard, Guy.
    [Audition égale comportement. English]
    Hearing equals behavior / Guy Bérard.
      p.   cm.
    Includes bibliographical references and index.
    ISBN 0-87983-600-8 : $17.95
    1. Hearing disorders—Psychological aspects. 2. Hearing impaired—Mental health. 3. Hearing disorders—Treatment—Case studies. 4. Mentally ill—Rehabilitation—Case studies. I. Title.
RF291.B47   1993
617.8′001′9—dc20   93-16937
                                        CIP

Printed in the United States of America

Published by Keats Publishing, Inc.
27 Pine Street (Box 876)
New Canaan, Connecticut 06840-0876

CONTENTS

ACKNOWLEDGMENTS

THIS TRANSLATION of Dr. Bérard's *Audition Égale Comportement* has been brought into being by many people who felt that Guy Bérard's important work should be available in English.

It started in California with Sandra and Howard Schlereth, whose autistic son Matthew showed remarkable improvement after treatment by Dr. Bérard. The Schlereths, wanting to better understand the process that had helped their son, engaged the services of Simone Monnier-Clay, who provided the first draft of the translated manuscript.

In the Midwest, Betty Mauzey refined the Simone Monnier-Clay translation for limited distribution to interested people at the Judevine School.

Meanwhile, in New York, Catherine Dodge, whose three learning-disabled children had all benefited from Dr. Bérard's auditory training, undertook the final reworking and editing of the translated manuscript primarily for distribution to students enrolled in the auditory training courses for practitioners, taught in Connecticut by Dr. Bérard under arrangement with the Georgiana Organization.

Thus the translation of *Audition Égale Comportement* which forms the core of the present book is the result of the combined efforts of a number of dedicated people.

Annabel and Peter Stehli, through the Georgiana Organization, arranged for the actual publication of the book by the Keats Publishing Company.

PREFACE

WHAT A PLEASURE it is for me, at last, to introduce this
English translation of Guy Bérard's *Audition Égale Comportement* to the numerous people it may help, but to whom it
was not previously accessible in its original French.

The English edition is the product of well over a decade
of joint effort by Dr. Bérard and numerous parents of
handicapped children, including myself. As Director of the
Autism Research Institute in San Diego, I had for many
years been investigating various forms of therapy for autistic children when I first learned of the work of Dr. Guy
Bérard, a little-known physician from a small town in a
remote area of France. Dr. Bérard was reportedly bringing
about significant improvement in a number of autistic children by having them listen to electronically altered music!
A strange way of trying to remedy a severe, life-long disability, I thought. An unlikely treatment from an unlikely
source.

But it was not easy to discredit the enthusiastic accounts
of the parents who, aware of my quest for better treatments
for autistic children, had written or phoned me, over a
period of years, to tell me of the exciting improvements
they had seen in their children. I was skeptical, but I did
not let my skepticism deter me from investigating the matter. In the mid-1960s I had been just as skeptical when I
first heard from a number of parents that they had seen
very significant improvement in their autistic children when
given high doses of certain vitamins, and had seen deterio-
ration in behavior when the vitamins were withdrawn. Set-
ting aside my skepticism, I initiated several experimental

studies and found, to my pleasure and surprise, that the parents were quite correct. The initial studies have been strongly confirmed. As of this writing (March, 1993) there have been 16 published experimental studies in 5 countries, showing that high doses of vitamin B6 and magnesium are helpful to nearly half of all autistic children and adults on whom they have been tried. No study has failed to demonstrate significant benefits, and no study has reported any significant adverse effects in any of the hundreds of patients on which the B6 and magnesium were tried. This is a far better record of safety and efficacy than exists for any drug. Nevertheless, despite the highly significant and consistent scientific findings, there is a great deal of skepticism from people who would rather doubt than look at evidence.

Thus, being very much aware that parental reports of improvement should not be lightly dismissed, I initiated correspondence with Dr. Bérard in the late 1970s, and invited him to visit me in San Diego in 1981.

Nothing came of his visit. The colleagues whom I had hoped to interest in Guy's work were polite, but not willing to collaborate in research. The same response—or lack of response—greeted my attempts, a year later, to stimulate interest by circulating several copies of this book, when it was first published, to scientists who could read French, and would presumably be interested in exploring promising treatments for autism.

Clearly, it seemed, this was an idea whose time had not come.

Enter Annabel and Peter Stehli and their daughter Georgie. No need to recount Georgie's story here—you will find it very well presented by Guy himself, and by Annabel, elsewhere in this book, and of course in Annabel's wonderful book *Sound of a Miracle*.

At last, in the mid-1980s, there was a way, it seemed, to get public and professional attention for Guy's work. Not only was Georgie's improvement—dare I say recovery—spectacular, but, in addition, it was obvious from Annabel's letters to me that she was a talented writer. It took a little persuasion, and encouragement to induce Annabel to undertake the writing of *Sound of a Miracle*, but once she got started, she proceeded with astonishing speed and skill. *Sound of a Miracle* deserved and received a great deal of favorable media attention.

When the *Reader's Digest* published an excerpted version of *Sound of a Miracle* in December, 1990, mentioning the name of our institute, our phone started ringing from morning till night, for many months. One father who finally reached us said that he had tried repeatedly for ten days before succeeding. "How can we get this treatment for our child" they all asked.

At first things were grim. Annabel was despondent—thousands of people were clamoring for auditory training for their children, and there was no way for them to get it. There were only two of Guy's electronic devices available in all of North America, and only two trained practitioners.

But, thanks to *Sound of a Miracle* and Annabel's tireless efforts, things have changed quickly. Now there are about 150 practitioners in various parts of the U.S. and Canada, and the number is growing.

"Does it really work?" I am asked that question repeatedly. "Yes," I reply. "I am reasonably certain that it does work." It will be several years before enough scientific evidence is in to permit categorical statements to be made, but judging from the evidence at hand, I feel, as does my colleague Dr. Stephen Edelson, who has been collaborating in research with me, that many, if not most, parents of autistic children who try Dr. Bérard's method will be justifiably pleased with the results.

Dr. Edelson and I recently completed a small-scale double blind experimental study on 17 autistic children in which significant differences were observed on several measures of improvement. We have collected data on a much larger sample, close to 400 subjects, and will soon be able to report the results. Further, other investigators have begun to conduct research on Auditory Integration Training, AIT as we now call it, in the U.S. and abroad, so it will not be long before a substantial body of scientific data is available on the effects of AIT on autistic persons.

But quite apart from the scientific data, Dr. Edelson and I, and Annabel, as you will read in her Afterword to this book, have heard from many hundreds of families whose children have undergone Bérard AIT. The vast majority of these people are pleased—and most are more than mildly pleased—with the changes in their children that they attribute to AIT. The reported changes are surprisingly diverse. Not just reduced sound sensitivity, but better attention span, better eye contact, more social awareness, fewer tantrums, more and better speech, and so forth. These and other changes are so consistently reported that it seems highly unlikely that it is merely wishful thinking. The high level of parent satisfaction is especially significant when one considers that their expectations, from having read of Georgie's improvement, were initially quite high.

Skeptical and cautious people warn us about placebo effects, of the danger of being deluded by wishful thinking. However autism is a poor field in which to expect strong placebo effects. Far from it—most autistic children are so refractory, and most changes that do occur take place so slowly, that Dr. Edelson and I believe the changes that are reported within days or months after undertaking AIT as being quite real, in most cases. We continue to be pleasantly surprised and optimistic.

It seems that the time for *this* idea has finally come.

B. Rimland, Ph.D.
Director, Autism Research Institute
San Diego
March 1993

INTRODUCTION

IT IS OBVIOUS that people who cannot hear well will experience difficulties in many aspects of life, and particularly that children who cannot hear clearly what the teacher is saying will be at a great disadvantage in school. In my practice as an otorhinolaryngologist—an ear, nose and throat specialist—I worked with many children whose hearing problems were affecting their school work, and came to see two important things.

One was that there was a direct rather than an indirect connection between poor hearing and disruptive classroom behavior. That is, it is a common assumption that the child who can't hear well becomes frustrated and bored, and because of this boredom and frustration "acts up." There is something to that, of course, but it became clear to me in the course of my work that hearing problems had a much more direct effect on behavior, and later work and tests confirmed this.

The other major discovery concerned the nature of the hearing problems affecting behavior. Traditionally, hearing is regarded as ranging from "good" to "bad," from being "able to hear a pin drop" to being extremely "hard of hearing," and hearing function tests are performed from this point of view. However, it became evident that there were variations in hearing dysfunction, and that either abnormal sensitivity or abnormal insensitivity to certain frequencies—rates of vibration—of sound waves, independently of overall hearing ability, were clearly associated with many behavior and learning problems, including hyperactivity and dyslexia.

I devised a technique of auditory training, in effect a "reeducation" of the hearing mechanism, which in almost every case brought about the normalization of the response to the frequencies involved—and, almost always, the amelioration of the behavior or learning problem.

To claim to have cured hyperactivity or dyslexia, widely regarded as "emotional" or "mental" conditions, simply by training the ear to be either more or less responsive to particular sound frequencies seems on the face of it implausible and extravagant. However, thirty years of clinical work, research and follow-up on more than 2,100 patients, and study of more than 8,000 auditory cases, verifies the claim. Of the 1,850 learning/behavior problems patients, three-quarters showed very positive results and the remainder demonstrated noticeable partial improvement; *none* failed to show some benefit. Many more patients have been treated since then, but the percentages of improvement have remained identical.

As the work progressed, I found that two more "emotionally" based problems appeared to be related to this type of hearing dysfunction. One, which has occasioned a great deal of publicity, and in fact led to the establishment of the Georgiana Organization, which is facilitating the publication of this book in the United States, is autism, that still-mysterious condition in which a person becomes a "prisoner inside himself," severely limited in his or her ability to communicate with others and apparently uninterested in doing so. The complete cure of Georgiana Stehli, narrated in Annabel Stehli's *The Sound of a Miracle*, is the most spectacular success with this condition. None of the 47 other autistic patients I treated up to 1982 achieved this level of success, but all did experience some improvement, many regaining the ability to speak or developing it for the first time; since that time I have been able with later patients to experience very important improvement, up to 90 percent.

The other "emotional" condition, suicidal depression, provides perhaps a more remarkable, certainly a more encouraging, story. I shall describe the discovery of the hearing-depression link in Chapter 3, and need here say only that 93 percent of the 233 patients treated for this condition were cured after the first course of auditory training, and 4.7 percent were healed after two or three courses.

In this book I shall explain how I arrived at the auditory training approach for these conditions and how I applied them, as well as showing how to determine if an individual's behavior problems are caused by hearing problems, and demonstrating the nature of the auditory training process and the apparatus used for both testing and training. I shall also discuss the nature of the hearing process and of the particular hearing disorders I deal with here, and offer some speculations on why it is that they affect behavior as they appear to do. I must emphasize that such speculations can be no more than preliminary, and hope that future research will provide definite answers in this remarkable and important area.

PART ONE

Background and Practice of
Auditory Training

Chapter 1

HEARING AND HEARING PROBLEMS

HEARING IS the perception of sound, and includes both the physical reception of the sound and its encoding and transmittal as information to the brain.

When we are hearing well, we receive the full range of sounds around us and can interpret them accurately, even when there are many sound sources present at the same moment. We can listen to a friend talking while music is playing, a dog is barking, traffic noises drift in from outside, and a faucet is slowly dripping in another room, and without effort understand the nature of each of these sounds and pay attention to those we consider important.

If you record a conversation in which you are a participant, then play it back, you are often surprised at the amount of background noise interfering with the talkers. The tape recorder performs the first function of hearing, registering the sound vibrations, but does not encode and select those requiring attention and "tuning out" the others, as we do in hearing.

The kind of hearing problem with which we are most familiar is a straightforward loss of the ability to hear sounds of low intensity—one becomes "hard of hearing" and turns the radio or TV louder, asks others to "speak up" and often requires a hearing aid. This is a simple deficiency in reception ability, and is compensated for by increasing the intensity, the loudness, of the sound by one means or another.

The problems I shall discuss in this book are a good deal more complex and little understood, and, as I hope to show, have remarkable effects upon behavior. Though mechanical in origin, as is the condition of being "hard of hearing," they profoundly affect the encoding and decoding operations of hearing, and therefore result in the brain receiving garbled information, not simply diminished information.

The keystone of this book and of the treatment I describe in it is my observation, based upon clinical experience of thousands of cases, that *everything happens as if human behavior were largely conditioned by the manner in which one hears.* Keep this in mind as you read, for what I suggest about the cause and treatment of behavior problems depends completely upon it.

I will start by discussing briefly the anatomical and physiological elements involved in the transmission of sound and its reception, both normal and abnormal. These are

> the sound stimulus
> the anatomical system and its function
> the failings of this system

THE SOUND STIMULUS

Sound is an atmospheric vibratory phenomenon, the physical vibration of the particles of the gases that compose the air that surrounds us. An object that is made to vibrate rapidly, for example by an impact, transmits those vibrations to the air, and if they reach an eardrum or microphone before fading out, they are received as sound. The schoolbook drawing of a stone being dropped in water sending out concentric circles of waves, which are larger closer to the point of impact and diminish as they move away from that point, is a simplified but valid illustration of the process. As with the ripples on the water, the vibrations pass through the air; they push a mass of air from the sound's point of origin to the perceiving, or hearing, organism.

There are two main characteristics of sound waves, frequency and amplitude. Amplitude refers to the power with which the waves are transmitted, which is registered by the ear as varying degrees of loudness. The units of measure of loudness are called decibels (abbreviated dB, and named for Alexander Graham Bell, the inventor of the telephone), ranging from the rustling of leaves at 20 dB to a rock band at 120 dB or more. The decibel scale is logarithmic, so that 10 dB is ten times as powerful as 1 dB, 20 dB is a hundred times as powerful, and 100 dB is 10 *billion* times as powerful.

Hearing is most often described as good or bad according to the level of decibels the person perceives; if your ear will not register an amplitude of less than 30 dB, you will not hear a friend a few feet away whispering to you, and if the lower limit is much higher than 60 dB, hearing ordinary conversation will be extremely difficult.

Hearing problems, then, as mentioned above, are usually considered to be a matter of amplitude, and devices, such as hearing aids, that mechanically or electronically amplify the sound waves received are the most common solution. The hearing difficulties which I have observed to be related to the types of behavior I have mentioned involve the other principal characteristic of sound, frequency.

Reasonably enough, this term refers to the number of vibrations transmitted in a given period. It is measured in vibrations per second, and the unit of measure is the hertz (Hz, named for the physicist Heinrich Hertz); 500 Hz denotes 500 vibrations, or cycles, per second.

Sound as humans perceive it falls in the range between 15 Hz and 20,000 Hz (sometimes written as 20 kilohertz or 20 kHz); to us, these are the "audible" frequencies. Vibrations below this level are referred to as infrasound; above it as ultrasound. Ultrasound is employed in "silent" dog whistles, which allow the whistler to transmit noises in excess of 20 kHz which he cannot hear but to which his dog's more sensitive ears respond.

Frequency is experienced as pitch, from deep to high, or

from the lowest bass notes to well past the scope of any soprano.

Of course, the sound spectrum we perceive varies according to the individual, and there are those who can hear silent dog whistles or the sub-bass of a kettledrum that has almost ceased to vibrate. For this book we shall ignore such exceptional cases and focus on the area most often perceived, between 125 Hz and 8,000 Hz. These are the frequencies of human speech.

THE ANATOMICAL SYSTEM AND ITS FUNCTION

Our hearing apparatus is composed of three elements:

the external ear
the middle ear
the internal ear

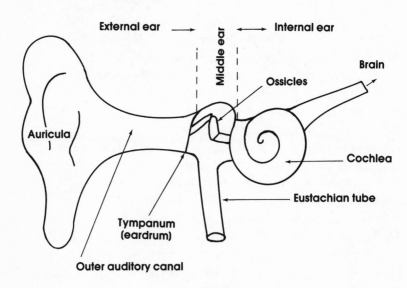

FIGURE 1-1

The external ear is the ear we all see, which some of us adorn with earrings, which others tape to the side of the head to train not to protrude, which we cup with our hands to focus faint sounds. This shallow convoluted cup of skin and cartilage is called the auricula, and is the first point of interception of sound waves. The narrow neck of this funneling apparatus is the outer auditory canal, which guides the sound vibrations to the eardrum, which forms the outer boundary of the middle ear.

The eardrum is also called the tympanum, from the Greek word for "drum." While an actual drumhead produces sound vibrations upon being struck, the eardrum vibrates in response to the sound vibrations it receives. Its upper portion is attached to an ossicle ("little bone") called the hammer, which is connected to the other ossicles, the anvil and the stirrup; all these are named for their shapes.

These three ossicles make up an articulated system of levers which act like a piston to transmit the vibration of the eardrum to the fluid in the cochlea, a spiral structure in the inner ear. The middle ear also contains the eustachian or auditory tube, which connects to the pharynx, the passage that connects the mouth and nasal cavity with the larynx. This structure, scarcely an eighth of an inch in diameter, equalizes air pressure on both sides of the eardrum. (You make conscious use of the eustachian tube when you swallow to relieve pressure in your ears on an airplane flight or after a swift elevator ride.) If the air pressure is not equal, the eardrum cannot vibrate properly, and hearing is impaired.

The inner ear is an extremely complex structure, of which for our present purposes it is enough to say that its role is to transform the vibratory energy of sound into nervous energy. The mechanical energy impinging on the cochlea is converted to activity of the auditory nerve fibers, which transport information to those sections of the brain that will decode it. The inner ear is the organ of perception, in contrast to the middle ear, the organ of transmission.

The auditory retraining methods I discuss in this book are directed at improving or normalizing the function of several parts of the ear:

the eardrum, because as the low-frequency sounds are working on the lower part of the drum, the high frequencies strike the upper part, and the combination amounts to a mechanical massage of this membrane the middle ear, specifically the eardrum;

the ossicles, by moving their joints, with the joint of the stirrup bone moving in the oval window like a piston;

the cochlea, as each part of the cochlea corresponds to one frequency, the high frequencies being located close to the oval window and the low frequencies in the middle of the spiral, you obtain another massage, probably through the cochlear liquid and perhaps through blood circulation.

FAILINGS OF THE SYSTEM

There are many obstacles that can affect the flow of sound from its inception at the outer ear to its decoding in the brain.

Vibration is a physical phenomenon, and interference with its reception will mainly be caused by mechanical problems.

• Total or partial obstruction of the external auditory canal. Ear wax, or the presence of a foreign body—a piece of cotton, a bread crumb, a pearl or a pencil tip, or a grain of wheat starting to sprout—are enough to reduce the sound stimulus by many decibels. An infection of the canal, external otitis (inflammation of the ear) or a polyp or other growth could have the same effect.

• Eardrum problems. It can be thickened or affected by eczema, or even torn. Its mobility can be hampered by the presence of excess liquid or pus in the inner ear or by defective functioning of the eustachian tube, so that air pressure is not equal on both sides.

• Malfunctioning of the ossicles. Their movement can be blocked by interior otitis or the presence of sclerous (hardened) tissue, or a genetic defect can fuse the anvil and stirrup. Any alteration in the middle ear reduces the transmission of incoming sound.

All these mechanical obstructions to the flow of sound can be treated appropriately, with a very good chance of success:

• The auditory ducts can be cleared by cleaning or localized treatments.

• Damaged eardrums can be rebuilt.

• Medical treatments such as thermal treatment or surgery can deal with malfunctions of the middle ear.

In recent years considerable progress has been made, and some spectacular successes obtained, in the area of surgery for deafness, which primarily relates to the middle ear. Problems of the inner ear are much more complex and difficult to deal with.

For instance, if the cochlea has been affected by hereditary factors, by a circulatory problem or by side effects of medication, the prognosis is less clear, and the chance of sound being allowed to reach the brain unimpaired is reduced.

Accidental severing of the auditory nerve will result in a total and permanent loss of hearing on the side affected. There are also cases, fortunately quite rare, of compression of this nerve by a cystic tumor; these, if diagnosed early enough, can be satisfactorily resolved through surgery.

The destruction, by disease or injury, of auditory brain cells will also affect hearing negatively.

HEARING TESTS AND WHAT THEY SHOW

To determine to what extent and in what manner hearing may be impaired, it must, of course, be tested. Here is a brief survey of the tests most frequently in use during the time I was in active practice.

• Pure-tone audiogram. This will be discussed in detail later; here it is enough to say that it tests response to both sound frequencies, from 125 Hz to 8000 Hz, and levels of intensity, transmitted by an instrument called the audiometer.

• The vocal audiogram, testing the comprehension of words.

• The tympanogram, which uses pressure to measure the functioning of the eardrum.

• The electrocochleogram, which measures the electric current generated by the cochlea.

• The Bekesy test; this is semi-automatic measurement of auditory function at all frequency levels.

• The Sisi test, which measures unusually low tolerances for particular frequencies, resulting in pain when these frequencies are experienced; this phenomenon is called "recruitment."

• The peep-show, an audiometric procedure for children of 3 or 4, using a toy train.

• Measurement of auditorily evoked potentials, by which is meant the electrical responses in the brain to stimuli from the cochlea.

Close study of test results, together with careful questioning and other radiological or laboratory examinations, allows the examiner to establish just how much hearing loss the patient is experiencing and just which area of the hearing apparatus is affected. One can then suggest to the patient what sort of solution would be appropriate: surgery, medicine or prosthesis—that is, hearing aids.

These tests are more important than most people realize, as it is estimated that 5 percent to 10 percent of persons in developed countries suffer some form of hearing impairment, which in most cases cannot be adequately diagnosed, and in many cases would not even be recognized, without such testing.

QUALITATIVE AND QUANTITATIVE TESTING

As I have said, quantitative problems of hearing are the most familiar ones to us: how well we pick up sounds as they become less intense, or fainter. The observations in this book will deal mainly with the qualitative aspects of hearing: with what level of distortion-free accuracy the vibrations striking the ear are received and decoded in the brain. To measure these aspects I have refined the testing procedure to produce a more precise audiogram.

There is no conflict between attending to the quantitative and to the qualitative components of hearing; in fact, they complement each other. The standard auditory quotient, the measurement used to indicate hearing efficiency, involves both the quantitative and qualitative aspects, and is arrived at by averaging test results of sound transmitted at three frequency levels (500 Hz, 1,000 Hz and 2,000 Hz). If the intensity required for the subject to perceive these frequency levels averages 15 decibels for the three, the auditory quotient is 100 percent.

The more precise audiogram I use in my work measures reception of sound transmitted at *all* frequencies, providing a full-spectrum profile of the subject's hearing.

I shall describe in detail in Chapter 5 both the standard quantitative tests and the qualitative tests which I have developed.

EYES AND EARS

We are used to problems of vision being complex and varied, and it is necessary to realize that hearing problems are far more so than we have been aware of.

Between the extremes of perfect visual acuity and total blindness, the eye can display many abnormalities: myopia, astigmatism, presbyopia, hypermetropia, divergent or convergent strabismus and so on. These conditions disturb the reception and decoding of the light signals entering the eye, and the affected person sees something other than what is objectively present. Most such problems are readily dealt with by the use of appropriate corrective lenses.

We are, therefore, quite used to eyeglasses. If a child must nearly bury his nose in a book to read it, we know that he sees poorly. He is taken to an ophthalmologist and given a prescription for the appropriate glasses; the child quickly gets used to the glasses and has a much easier time of it in school.

Yet problems of hearing, other than evident degrees of deafness, are by no means as well understood, and are often ignored or even denied. The reason for this is that evidence of such hearing dysfunction is not as obvious as it is for visual dysfunction. Visual perception deals with objects which both are definite and possess duration—they may be observed for a distinct period of time, and one individual's perception of them can be compared in detail with another's. In case of any difficulty in making the comparison, all the time necessary can be taken; the data are stable.

It is very much different with auditory problems. The sounds which reach our ears are fleeting, fluctuating, constantly changing. (Continuous loud sounds, such as heavy machinery, are an exception to this statement, but not one which affects its general application.) In a conversation between two people, one cannot establish the perception each had of the same sound. Was it louder for one than for the other? Lower pitched? No comparison can be established, for the sound perceived is gone, replaced by a multitude of succeeding sounds.

Hearing problems are therefore more complex and less perceptible in everyday life; and in fact they can be satisfactorily diagnosed and defined only through systematic tests of the kind briefly noted above.

In the next chapter I shall explore the effects of hearing on behavior, mainly in children and particularly the problems brought about by hearing abnormalities.

Chapter 2

HEARING AND BEHAVIOR

I REPEAT HERE the key statement I made in the first chapter: *Everything happens as if human behavior were largely conditioned by the manner in which one hears.* Now it is time to amplify that and, if needed, persuade the reader of its truth.

Starting with birth—even *in utero,* some people believe—the individual is continuously in an environment of sound. This constant bath of sound is passed from the external ear to the middle ear and finally to the inner ear, from where it is transmitted to the auditory center in the brain.

What does this incessant flow of sound information bring to the individual?

In his development, possibly even before his birth, sound teaches him about his environment. First he learns, then recognizes, specific sounds related to his needs or fears: endearing voices or angry ones, abnormal noises which startle him. Later comes the understanding of phenomena, including the imitation of those phonemes and elementary musical notes which began with lullabies. The perfection of this learning process and conditioning to sound proceeds, accompanied by the acquisition of an increasingly elaborate vocabulary, which leads to real speech. The child blossoms toward a perfected language, toward passive music (listening), then active music (singing), and at last, instrumental music.

ENVIRONMENT, HEALTH AND BEHAVIOR

The personal environment of each person is made up of his or her family and social and professional circles. To these each of us brings our own personality, a personality formed by our unique physical, psychological and intellectual traits, and our behavior exhibits a profile determined by that personality.

Now let an event occur powerful enough to alter one or more elements in the personality, and the behavior profile alters accordingly. If someone close dies, if there is a birth, if you are promoted at work, or demoted or fired, there will be an impact on your personality and your behavior will be affected: the joyful, optimistic component of your personality will be enhanced or diminished.

The people who share your life will notice the change and tell each other, if not you, that you are "not the same"—happier than before, more depressed than before, but not the same as before.

And yet you are the same—the same "global" individual, but changed in behavior by the circumstances of your life.

With physical problems, this is even more evident. The person living with chronic pain, even of the mild, "nagging" kind, will eventually show it. He may bear it without obvious complaint, but being stoic about pain is in itself different behavior from living pain-free. Even if there is no obvious injury, those around him will see a change.

And pain can affect behavior even more directly and obviously. Someone who enjoys participating in sports who develops a joint pain such as bursitis or arthritis can no longer do this and will have to adjust his life and activities accordingly. He will no longer be the person he was, in his own view and that of those around him.

I have said nothing here that is not fully obvious, but I wish to have these concepts in the forefront of the reader's mind as we progress.

Consider next defects of vision. In these, evidence of changed behavior is also clear. When vision problems develop, the first effects are usually minor inconveniences, such as fatigue while driving, particularly at night, headaches during reading, and apprehension when lights are excessively bright or dim. If the problems become worse, vision of every sort will become uncertain. Even the minor problems affect personality and conduct, for example promoting indecisiveness and uncertainty. This personality change can be almost totally reversed with correct treatment of the visual deficit, usually with corrective lenses, and the person will be virtually his "old self" (except of course for having a pair of glasses resting on the bridge of his nose). If the visual problems appear in childhood, they are generally diagnosed and treated quickly, and the glasses become part of the physical-psychosocial persona of the child and the adult into whom the child grows.

HEARING DISTORTION

This is the heart of the problem. Let us begin with some general observations before going into detail.

Let us consider a person functioning satisfactorily in every way, and then let us interfere with his hearing. If we make him totally deaf, we expect that his behavior will be radically disturbed, and we will find it easy to see why this would be so, and that it would be true even of somewhat less severe hypacousia (a drop in hearing ability).

But now suppose that our subject experiences painful hearing in the high frequencies, say when presented with a sound with an intensity of 40 dB at and above a frequency of 2,000 Hz.

What happens? The subject will find these sounds unpleasant and threatening, and will try to avoid hearing them: avoiding suffering is a high-priority activity for any organism.

What are the sources of such sounds? There are a great many, including people with high voices, some music, noises from loudspeakers in the street, and children's playtime screams; and this list barely scratches the surface of the list of traumatizing sounds in this intensity-frequency range.

Imagine our poor subject, married, say, to a soprano and employed as a building contractor. At the end of a day of screeching machinery on the job, he returns home to a volley of high C's from his diligently practicing wife, to ear-piercing shrieks of delight from the smaller children and to the latest style of music pounding out from his eldest son's stereo.

The main social, familial and professional consequences are clear. The subject will go to work with anticipatory anguish, will return home with apprehension and will arrange his movements to avoid the dreaded levels of noise as much as possible. He may well turn away from society and as a result be labeled abnormal and antisocial, or possibly be stigmatized as psychotic or semi-psychotic. If he or those close to him are disturbed enough by what is happening to him, he may be funnelled into psychiatric treatment, which without doubt will do him no good.

But a well-administered audiometric examination could make clear precisely what his problem is. And when its nature is established, that problem is often readily solvable, as I shall show later.

DEFECTIVE HEARING IN CHILDREN

In the rest of this chapter I shall deal with learning disabilities in children and the role hearing plays in them. (In France the term "dyslexia" is used to denote these problems, including but not limited to the specific difficulty with reading so called in the United States. I shall use it in the way I am most accustomed to, but will point out where relevant any information bearing on the condition as it is understood in the U.S.)

We will look at what can happen when a child experiences defective hearing that is neither deafness nor a less intense hypacousia.

Children as young as a few months of age are already receptive to the sounds of their environment. How they perceive sounds becomes increasingly important as they acquire language skills. And any abnormality in verbal perception will result in an inaccurate imitation of the sound. When the child goes to school, serious difficulties will develop. At home a parent might be amused by a mispronunciation, and be willing to accommodate to a child's slowness in comprehension or reaction by taking the time to repeat a word until it is understood. At school it is different. The child is immersed in a new society, in a situation by no means set up to accommodate him. The teacher will speak at a normal pace and will use new words which will need to be repeated, sorted and registered in the child's memory.

Let us imagine, for instance, a child suffering from an auditory *dyslaterality*. I shall discuss laterality and dyslaterality in detail later on but it is enough for now to say that dyslaterality is a condition in which sounds of certain frequencies are perceived by one ear and not the other, or more weakly by one than by the other. A lack of laterality results in an inversion in the perception of certain letters or groups of letters—we will find out why that is so in the detailed discussion. For example, if the teacher says "cob," the child may hear "bock" or perceive "cool" as "look."

When listening to the teacher, such a child does not comprehend the whole word first, but unconsciously yet permanently organizes the perceived phonemes—basic sounds—in a specific order. He will then put each word in its place beside the others, and only when the whole phrase has been "heard" in this manner can the child's intelligence operate to grasp the sense of the phrase and the message it contains.

This cumbersome process is difficult and time-consuming. Some words will be "heard" wrong; others will be slowly sorted out correctly. The child will be at a loss compared with his classmates. He will have been penalized by time, because it takes him longer to understand, and handicapped by the fatigue caused by the extra effort. However willing, he may not be able to sustain the full class hour. He may remain attentive and alert for fifteen minutes or half an hour, but then his attention will wander. After a time of this, school will seem a burden and the remainder of the term will stretch ahead like a prison sentence. Early enthusiasm and excitement, spurred by the parents' encouragement, will give way to apathy or revolt, according to the child's temperament.

Then what happens?

In the worst cases, fortunately also the rarest, the parents and teachers lose interest in the matter and the child falls behind in classwork. He is repeatedly punished, and tries to affirm himself in ways that are not productive. He may become disruptive or bullying; he may get into mischief and lie to conceal it. He may start to skip classes, then go on to reject school totally. His whole school career may be seriously jeopardized, with grave consequences for the rest of his life.

Most of the time, the parents and teachers agree that "something isn't right" and get together to find out what is bothering the child. They discuss earnestly the question of whether the child is making an effort. Does he understand what is expected of him? If not, why? Is that the problem or is it something else entirely?

It is soon clear that there are no immediate useful answers, and the search begins. First the pathological option is explored. The doctor examines the child and orders a variety of lab tests; the ophthalmologist finds or does not find eye problems. Sometimes a treatable condition is found and everyone's hopes are raised, but the situation does not improve.

Our student is now referred to the school psychologist. With the parents' help, the psychologist gathers all possible information on the manifest problem and anything that might be related to it in the child's life, and administers tests and makes evaluations necessary to creating a psycho-intellectual profile of the child.

And all of these tests will always show a deficit in a given area, because the child is not functioning normally. Equipped with this information, the psychologist directs the child, depending on the findings, toward psychotherapy, speech therapy, treatment dealing with behavior disorders, or treatments meant to remedy dyslexia—for my American readers, learning disability.

There, we have said the word. Yes, madam, your child is learning-disabled.

And now we have this poor mother looking for information about this new epidemic. Her sisters—other mothers of dyslectic/learning-disabled children—will suggest what might be tried, based on their own experience. Libraries, bookstores and magazines offer a wide variety of explanations and theories, some so complex as to set the parents wondering about possible learning disabilities of their own. At this point they can consider themselves lucky if no one suggests that they themselves are responsible for the child's condition. This is a good deal less common than it used to be some decades ago, when it was fashionable to blame parents for everything distressing to or about their children, but it happens occasionally, and when it does, it is a needless addition to the burden of dealing with the child's problem.

And now let us return to the ear. What role does it play in all this?

Has science not thought, not wanted to think of, or simply neglected to think of the fact that the child must first understand a question in order to answer it correctly? To understand, the child must *hear the question as it was asked*, without the need of a constant effort to perceive and arrange the exact words. Any of us who has learned a foreign language has experienced something of this effort when listening to a more fluent speaker of the language: we snatch at the words as they come by, try to hear and understand and link to the ones before and after. If we mistake even one word, the sense of the whole sentence may be lost. And then consider the case of a child to whom every conversation in his own language presents the same problem.

As long as this basic fact is not recognized, diagnostic testing cannot be effective. Unless the cornerstone of examination of auditory function is in place, the whole structure of diagnosis is unstable. If the child's auditory integrity is compromised, all other tests will be invalid; i.e., no answer to a question is indicative of a level of mental acuteness *if the question is not heard correctly*. A parallel can be drawn with the situation of giving a child with myopia a written test for mental function without allowing the use of glasses: it would clearly be absurd to arrive at any judgments in such

21

a circumstance, except perhaps of the wisdom of the test givers.

After I came to see and accept this concept, I conducted a study to verify it, using several children with a variety of "dyslexias." The first stage, before even the audiometric examination, was a series of simple tests to establish mental age, I.Q. and a psychological profile.

After this, a standard ear, nose and throat, or ENT, examination was done, and then audiometric testing. Treatment was determined by the results of these procedures: medical, surgical or—the main treatment discussed in this book—retraining of the ear.

If the treatment decided on was retraining, twenty half-hour sessions were given at the rate of two a day, and another audiogram was done to see what the retraining had accomplished. Usually the hearing defect had been completely or substantially relieved. The day following the second audiogram, we gave a second series of the tests given at the outset to show what the child was like intellectually and psychologically. We were surprised (at first; later we came to expect it) to find that, when the hearing was normalized, the mental age rose by an average of from 1 to 2 years and the I.Q. gained from 10 to 15 points over the earlier values.

Obviously, no child becomes substantially more intelligent in just ten days. What clearly happened is that the children's newly normalized hearing allowed them to use a great deal more of their intellectual potential.

It is only when hearing is known beyond doubt to be normal, preferably by testing, that the testing to evaluate I.Q., mental age and psychological profile should be done. Only then will the test results have validity and meaning and the conclusions derived be valid. Let me repeat, because it is so important and so disregarded, that no test can be reliable if the child "hears wrong" while he is taking the test.

Does this mean that every instance of dyslexia or learning disability is related to hearing? Of course not. But it now appears vital that any hearing anomaly, no matter how minimal, in a child experiencing difficulty in school should be closely looked into. If hearing dysfunction is found, that problem must be treated before doing anything else. In fact, in my experience, very nearly all children with dyslexia or other learning disabilities display one or more hearing anomalies upon undergoing thorough hearing examinations.

I conducted a different study which bore out this concept from the other direction. We did anonymous audiometric testing of students from the same class or the same family, with no somatic examination and no questions that might have unconsciously affected administration of the tests. The results showed clearly that the children who received the best grades in class and demonstrated the most satisfactory behavior were all endowed with hearing free of any major abnormality.

We did find a few students with a degree of hearing dysfunction who did extremely well in school, but parents and teachers told us that these showed a strong will to work and put more time and effort into school work than the average student. This allowed these students to compensate for their hearing deficit, as they might compensate in a sport where rigorous training and a strong will can out-weigh some physical deficiency. President Theodore Roosevelt is often offered as an example of this.

AUDITORY ABNORMALITIES, DISTURBANCES AND LEARNING DISABILITIES

I have found in the course of my work eight major types of abnormality in hearing which are implicated in behavior problems in children. Most of these are disclosed by the qualitative audiometric test I have developed; I shall point out any which are not. This list is probably not complete, and others will be discovered later on.

These abnormalities will be discussed fully in Chapter 5, which examines the testing procedures in great detail; here I shall describe them only sufficiently to explain their effect on learning and behavior.

1. Problems in response timing

With a normal subject, the "yes" indicating the perception of a sound and the "no" indicating its interruption take place within one second. In some cases the reaction time can be two or more seconds (sometimes, though rarely, up to five seconds). If, in the optimum conditions of quiet and concentration prevailing during the test it takes a child three seconds to take in one sound, it is easy to imagine what happens in a classroom with a spate of unknown words at a rate of several per second. A considerable effort of will may allow the child, for a while, to gather the information received and use it when needed. But it is soon overwhelmed, and then fatigue and errors arise, and so do reprimands.

"You see that you can do well when you try, since your last page was perfect. But now you do not care about your work. You have made a mistake with a word you wrote correctly before."

What can the child say to this? Nothing, since he does not have the key to the problem. No more than the teacher does, for that matter.

I should note here that school work in France involves a great deal more writing down of material dictated by the instructor than is the case in the United States, so that problems like that just described often become evident sooner and more clearly. But the problem exists everywhere to, I would guess, about the same extent.

2. Errors

The subject, particularly a child, can make several kinds of mistakes during the test, mainly either neglecting to indicate hearing a sound until some time after it is heard, or through overeagerness signaling hearing of a sound when none is being transmitted.

3. Fatigue

Fatigue has much the same effect as problems in response timing.

4. Painful hearing

If painful hearing is present, it is always found in the high frequencies. Although it usually begins at 4,000 Hz, we have been able to identify it as early as 1,500 Hz.

What is the result of painful hearing? First of all, the common-sense reactions. The child will look for quiet places; and it is important to note that he unconsciously selects the people who speak to him. He prefers the company of adults to that of children, and he feels more at ease surrounded by males than by females, whose voices are higher.

This is not as inconsequential as it might seem. Why does the child prefer a male teacher to a female: Why are his grades better in courses taught by a man than in those taught by a woman? The answer is not psychological, as is so often assumed, but physical, as we can find by asking the child: "Because I do not like Miss ———'s voice." Why would he like it if it hurts him? This answer is always given when an audiometric examination points to painful hearing.

Here is a typical case.

Before doing his own testing, a child psychologist sent a ten-year-old boy to me for auditory testing. The child had been having problems in school and with relationships.

The boy arrived accompanied by his father and mother. From the beginning of the session I noticed that the child, seemingly unaware of doing so, stayed closer to his father. Whatever the father said brought a nod or a smile from his son. All the explanations given by the mother were met with a frown, objections or a shrug. I asked when the child had his first ear infection; and, when the mother said it was when he was two, the child laughed and with a smirk proclaimed, "No, I was one!"

The somatic examination was completed without any problem, and we went into the audiology room, accompanied by the father, who said offhandedly, "Oh, you know . . . it's always the same at home—they argue constantly."

The audiogram started and the child answered perfectly on the frequencies of 125, 250, 1,000 and 1,500

Hz, each given with an intensity of 40 decibels, then progressively lowered all the way to the lowest level that could be heard.

When we tried the frequency of 2,000 Hz, the boy instantly tore off the headphone helmet being used and threw himself to the floor, screaming, "It hurts—like an electric shock!"

That alarmed me a little, because about two weeks previously I had in fact experienced an electric shock from different headphones, which had shaken me up a good deal. I knew that this could not happen with an audiometer, but . . . It seemed best to prove that there was no danger, and with considerable caution I put the earphones on to repeat the test, ready to expect anything. At the frequency of 2,000 Hz, I carefully began with 5 decibels and progressed to an output of 100 dB. Nothing happened.

I reassured the boy and went on with the examination, being careful to start transmission at the very low level of 5 dB, increasing the intensity progressively. And again, at 40 dB and 2,000 Hz, we reached the threshold that made the child cry; I could hardly calm him down. I then went on with the test in reverse, starting at the top of the scale with 8,000 Hz. Everything was calm until we reached the 2,000 Hz level and got the same response as before.

The solution to the problem with the child's mother was found! The parents, very positive people, saw it immediately, and the child confirmed it: "Yes, Mother's voice hurts my ears, and I prefer it when my father scolds me." The mother was unlucky enough to speak at a frequency of 2,000 Hz, precisely the frequency that so distressed her son.

The consultation, which had started so tensely, ended with joy. The distancing between mother and son was addressed immediately by the mother training herself to use a lower register when talking to him, and shortly solved permanently, along with the other behavior problems, by treating the child's hearing, which also had other abnormalities.

5. Auditory selectivity

Some people mishear frequencies in a drastic manner, hearing a tone of 6,000 Hz as higher than 8,000 Hz, or 500 Hz as the same as 1,000 Hz. Sometimes these distortions are spread evenly among the frequencies, and sometimes they occur in a range between two frequencies, with the area above and below them unaffected.

It is evident that a child who hears sounds going up the scale when they are in fact going down, or the other way round, will probably not like music, because he hears something other than what is presented to his ear. He will sing out of tune in spite of lessons. He will be unable to play any musical instrument except the piano, as, at least in the early stages, it requires mainly a purely mechanical involvement. The eyes reading the sheet music send out the information to the fingers, which in turn hit the keys, without any other form of control, manual or physical. At a more advanced technical level, however, the ear becomes necessary to control the sounds expressed. A child with this problem will not even want to consider taking up the profession of a violinist or orchestra conductor.

In fact, as soon as questioned, a child whose hearing is impaired in this way will usually say that he does not like music. As a rule we don't like anything we can't do easily, in work, in entertainment or in sport.

The problems in dealing with music are obvious and undeniable. But there is another level of problems. Spelling mistakes, especially in the area of "whistling words," can come from hearing that disturbs the child's perception—the child perceives "something else" than that which was a basic sound or harmony.

The gap can be more or less clear in a given language, but the picture clouds up considerably for some other languages. The range of frequencies used by each language varies, and it is evident that a child will have an easier time studying one that corresponds to his own selectivity.

In particular the study of Chinese, with its nine tones encompassing a maximum of frequencies and requiring attention and especially acute auditory precision, could not be taken on without problems. (With Chinese, the same monosyllabic phoneme can express nine different meanings, according to the chosen intonation.)

Here is an experience that illustrates this. It involves a university graduate with degrees in French and English, who now decided to undertake Italian studies. Brilliant as her written work was, she received surprisingly bad grades on the oral testing. Auditory testing revealed a trough at around 500 Hz, a frequency that corresponds to some specific inflections in the Italian language. Auditory training started right away and the trough disappeared. When we next met she told me she had passed her exams second among 250 candidates.

6. Auditory distortion

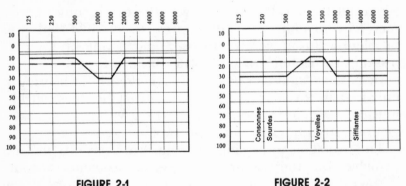

FIGURE 2-1   FIGURE 2-2

The audiograms illustrate this problem very clearly. The points located higher on the line indicate sounds that are better received than those that are lower, even though these sounds have been transmitted with identical intensities.

Figure 2-1 shows that if we transmit all the tones, from 125 Hz to 8,000 Hz, at a uniform intensity of 10 dB— shown by the broken straight line, the subject hears all frequencies *except* those of 1,000 and 1,500 Hz, which are located below the 10 dB line.

If we transmit at an intensity of 30 dB, the subject will

hear the 1,000 and 1,500 Hz tones, but more weakly than the others.

To illustrate how this bears on comprehension, and consequently behavior, we will use music as an example. When an orchestra accompanies a soloist, say a trumpeter, you follow the melody played by him note by note. The other instruments remain in the background; their purpose is to support the main theme. If the conductor does his job well, you do not notice the succession of notes coming from the violins or the brass; these are overshadowed by the notes of the soloist, even if those notes are not more important than those of the orchestra.

The same is true with a pianist: the principal theme will stand out from the total performance. The piano's melody will be heard over the less intense accompaniment.

In the area of speech—and therefore eventually in spelling—each group of letters of the alphabet, each phoneme, has a precise place in the audiometric diagram. We can say generally that the "hard" consonants (P, B, T, D, M, N, etc., designated CS in Figure 2-2) are located below 1,000 Hz, the "whistling" sounds (designated by S) are located above 1,500 Hz, and the vowels and diphthongs (V) are in between.

Figure 2-2 depicts the test of a child who perceived vowels and diphthongs most first, which tended to blur his hearing of the consonants. In everyday conversation this is rarely noticeable. If it is noticed, it seems so insignificant that an error in understanding a word seems to be absent-mindedness. However, in school, the instructor often speaks quickly and uses words new to the students, and the problem begins to have apparent effects. The child can write "bate" instead of "date" because he has not correctly heard the consonants "covered" by the sound of the vowel "a." The same problem can be found with "pike" and "bike," in which "p" and "b" could be covered by "i."

Figure 2-1 shows an opposite condition. The subject who has trouble differentiating in the 1,000-1,500 Hz zone may write "fowl" for "fool" or "curse" for "course."

It is possible to argue about the exact zone occupied by

each phoneme; scientists are not all in agreement about the placement of vowels and consonants on a frequency diagram. But this is not especially important for this discussion. The main point is that a tone better perceived at the purely auditory level will be better heard and recorded at the verbal level.

These two examples are typical and simplified, but you can find in a dyslexic/learning disabled child some or all of the complicated auditory abnormalities we discussed above, which produce the mistakes that the standardized educational and psychological tests do not explain.

There is an obvious objection to this contention: inconsistency in the mistakes. Why does the child sometimes write the "problem" word correctly and sometimes incorrectly? There are several excellent reasons for this. It can depend on the voice of the instructor, his pronunciation, and the rapidity of his use of phonemes. It can result from the child's individual auditory limitations, which either allow him to make or not make a correction regarding the phoneme he did not hear well.

If the child is doing a school exercise at home, he will make fewer mistakes because his parent will dictate according to his own speed, and usually close and face to face. In class the instructor talks to everyone, and not always face to face at the front of the classroom but from the sides of the room or with his back to the students. When during a child's audiometric examination we notice some important distortions of this sort, it is rare that the parents or the school work that is brought to us do not confirm this notion of localized errors in the area of auditory dysfunction.

What I have said applies to the French language, in which the frequency range used is well defined. But the reasoning remains valid for other languages, where sounds are placed differently. The observed audiometric abnormalities sometimes explain quite well why it is difficult to learn English, Italian or any other language. This problem of auditory anomalies may also be found with adults who want to study a foreign language later in life, but hit a wall in spite of their intelligence and hard work.

7. Auditory laterality

Discussing this topic is going to involve reviewing some basic anatamo-physiological concepts, starting with bilateral symmetry.

The human body consists of two halves which are pretty much "mirror images" of each other, the right side and the left side. The mobility of the body is controlled by the brain, and the central nerves cross over from one side to the other at the base of the skull. This means that each side of the body is dependent on the opposite side of the brain. The brain itself consists of two almost identical halves.

When you move your right index finger, the order for this movement is given by well-defined cells on the left side of the brain. You want to stretch your left leg? Other cells from the right brain will initiate your movement. This is easy enough to understand: left controls right, right controls left.

Now you wish to talk, and things are no longer so simple. The process is more involved because speech triggers an extremely complex mechanism. Drastically simplified, it involves:

a) the whole thoracic cavity and the diaphragm, which give to

b) the larynx the quantity of air needed to make the vocal cords vibrate. The sound produced will then be modified by

c) the cavum and inside of the mouth, where the action of the tongue is important in controlling internal vocal volume; and

d) the lips, which with their muscles allow movements of great diversity, and which have the task of giving the finishing touches to the sound produced.

But what coordinates this intricate sequence of actions of the muscles and nervous system involved in this process?

The center of speech is located in a well-defined location, almost always in the left brain. It consists of two areas called

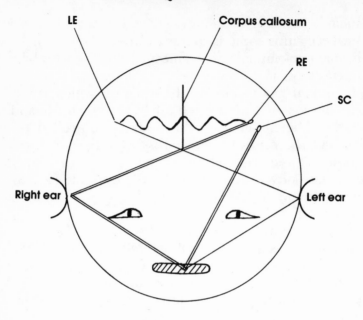

FIGURE 2-3

Broca's Area and Wernicke's Area, and is identified in Figure 2-3 by the letters SC.

What happens when we wish to formulate a sentence and set all this machinery moving? It will be necessary to control the output, the intensity and the sonority and, of course, the exactness of the spoken words. And what else than the brain can take over this constant checking?

When you talk, your hearing system tells you of the quality and of the exactness of your speech. Is your sound production too loud? Too weak? Your ear will notice immediately and will inform the speech center, which then makes the appropriate corrections.

Your ear, yes . . . but not just the either on any side!

Let us look at Figure 2-3 and see what takes place with one ear and then with the other.

First, assume the subject controls his speech with the right ear. The first syllable sent out by the mouth will spread into the air, but part of it will be gathered by the

32

right ear and sent to the auditory center located in the left brain (RE), since the nerves are crossed at the base of the skull. The whole circuit from mouth to right ear to left brain is almost instantaneous, a few milliseconds. The left brain cells of the right auditory system are very close to the brain area of speech to which they immediately give the information received.

The speech center SC continues to order the successive syllables, which are processed as they come from the mouth, in perfect chronological order, since a lapse of about 20/100 of a second takes place in regular speech output. The path from speech center to mouth to right ear to right ear perception is shown on the diagram by a double line.

Now let us suppose that our subject cannot hear on the right side. He will be forced to use his left ear to control his speech.

The circuit, the single line on the diagram, will be just as direct and fast as in the preceding case, up until LE, the auditory center for the left ear located in the right brain. Up to this point things have gone well, but now they become complicated. In order to get the incoming sound information to SC, the speech center, a barrier must be penetrated, the corpus callosum, the band of nerve fibers dividing the two halves of the brain. The absolute minimum necessary for this transfer of sound is estimated to be about 4/100 of a second, but this minimum is not the rule, it may take up to 40/100 of a second, sometimes even more.

What would be the consequence for this "left-eared" subject?

If the transfer time is 4/100 of a second, the effect on speech will be a minimal slowing down, not noticeable by the speaker.

However, as the length of the transfer time increases, the picture becomes darker. If we recall that the normal rate of speech corresponds to a syllable every 20/100 of a second, and that the next syllable cannot be processed until the one ahead has been checked, there will be a noticeable slowing of speech, with no indication of what causes it.

A theory of the mechanism of stuttering has been proposed, based on this left auditory laterality, with a delay in transmission of 20/100 of a second—that is the same as the elapsed time that normally separates two syllables—triggering a kind of echo of the preceding syllable, which is unconsciously repeated. It appears that some cases of stuttering definitely belong in this category.

It is possible to improve and sometimes to cure some of these speech difficulties by forcing the subject to use his right ear instead of his left. We can also create an artificial stuttering condition by transmitting a subject's voice only to his left ear, at the same time creating a 20/100 second delay; this reinforces the theory that that is how "natural" stuttering occurs.

Auditory lateralization to the right or the left is often associated with corporal lateralization, i.e. "handedness." We notice that most people who are totally "left-hearing" are also left-handed. The left ear is constantly at work. Everything happens as if the right cerebral auditory center, which is linked to the left ear, gets the information first, drawing to itself a larger blood supply. The neighboring nerve cells would benefit, and it is those cells that control the left limbs—remember, the nerves cross over, right brain to left side, left brain to right side, at the base of the skull.

And people who give priority to the right ear experience a more constant and active functioning of the left brain-right ear auditory center, with consequent hyperfunction of the neighboring cells and promotion of right-sidedness.

Here is an instance to illustrate this. We test a child whose body movements are poor, or not lateralized. He sits in a chair, with his legs swinging and with the earphones on his head. He is listening to music of a specific intensity transmitted alternately to the right and left ear. The subject is not distracted by anything else, and is being observed from a neighboring room.

In the majority of cases, after some time has elapsed, if we send sounds to the right ear only, we will see his eyes turn to the right, and the right leg will swing and the right hand will move to some extent. When we send the sound to the left ear only we will see the same motions on the left side.

After that rather technical excursion, let us see how all this applies in the school situation.

Up to now we have considered extreme conditions, presenting the problem as though everything takes place completely on the right or on the left. Things get more complicated when listening is alternated in a more random way, for example (again, a simplified one) when the subject hears the lower frequencies, up to 1,000 Hz, with the left ear and all others with the right ear.

If we recall that each group of letters occupies its own place in the frequency spectrum, we can see that the "hard" consonants (P,B,D,T, etc.) will be perceived with more or less delay in relation to vowels, diphthongs and "whistling letters." The level of comprehension necessary to learn new work or to take normal-speed dictation will decline. If the speech center receives information in a random manner, the letters cannot be placed in proper order and the message must be unscrambled before it is understood.

This explains the presence of the inversions of "classic" dyslexia. The subject writes the phonemes in the order in which he has *heard* them, but not in the order in which they were *presented* to him. Comparing audiograms with the type of mistake presented to us by parents confirms this observation.

Here again, these problems do not appear in everyday conversation, because the child has developed an automatic way of expressing himself, established by long experience and renewed every day. They also do not occur when dictation is slow, because the child has time to decode and correct any information that is garbled in reception.

As I have said, the examples I have presented have been simplified to make the basic idea clear. Exposing the ear to groups of phonemes at varying frequencies may indicate many more possible complications of hearing. The Weber test, in which varying frequencies are applied to the frontal bone, directly on the midline of the skull, can make clear the precise location and extent of problems with laterality. For this reason the examination must be done with the greatest care, cross-checking the answers several times in order to assure their accuracy.

Another abnormality can further complicate the problem of lateralization. You can demonstrate this yourself.

Cover your right ear with the palm of your hand. Count loudly, *One, two, three,* and so on. You will notice that your voice resounds in the right side of your head. You hear your own voice with your right ear. If you leave your hand covering the ear, you will notice that you hear outside sounds with your left ear. So you have one side of your brain or the other working, depending on whether someone is talking to you or you are doing the talking. This is a small complication.

This simple test lets us understand more completely what happens when a person is suffering from an impairment of hearing transmission. By that I mean a problem caused by a malfunction in the external ear or the middle ear. This happens with an individual who has one ear that functions perfectly and one that, even minimally, is affected by something that disturbs the transmission of sound. This can be ear wax, the presence of acute or chronic otitis, or poor permeability of the eustachian tube. In these cases the Weber test always locates the lateralization of sounds on the side on which transmission is poor.

The "small complication" grows enormously if, instead of the whole gamut of frequencies, the transmission blockage affects only some areas in either or both ears. The Weber test may show, for example, blockages in these areas:

right side	125 and 250 Hz
left	500, 1,000 and 1,500 Hz
right	2,000 Hz
left	4,000, 6,000 and 8,000 Hz

Knowing the location of the various letter groups in each frequency area, it is easy to imagine the gymnastics the brain must perform during a conversation or a dialogue, when the brain receives from the outside one set of phonemes from the right and another from the left . . . and with a delay! And on top of that, everything is inverted, even one's own speech! Definitely a major complication.

You can better understand the problem by drawing a parallel with sight. Try to read a book while closing each eye in turn for half a second. It may be possible to do this for a short space of time, but no longer.

8. Psychoneurotic aspect of responses.

This is, strictly speaking, not a matter of hearing, but of other factors affecting test responses. I shall discuss this in Chapter 5, which goes over all aspects of the testing procedure.

TO SUM UP

I hope I have demonstrated that each of the hearing abnormalities described here could negatively affect a child's experience and hence his behavior. An accumulation of deficiencies can only aggravate the situation.

When a child is brought to us by his parents and has fifty or sixty mistakes on one page of dictation, we know that the audiometric examination will systematically show the presence of several auditory deficiencies.

Chapter 3

DEPRESSION AND OTHER DISORDERS

MY MAIN FOCUS so far has been on children and how hearing problems affect their development and their school and social lives. Children grow into adults, and all too often uncorrected hearing dysfunction stays with them as they mature, causing old difficulties to persist and, sometimes, new ones to develop.

My own work led me to an astonishing discovery in this area, that a specific auditory deficiency is strongly linked to a very severe form of depression, and later in this chapter I shall discuss in detail how I determined this and what my experience has been in diagnosing and treating this condition. Before getting at this remarkable material, I must survey the matter of auditory dysfunction in adults in general.

COMPENSATING FOR HANDICAPS

When a child and his parents come to me for a consultation and the audiogram shows that a specific anomaly causes either learning disabilities or behavior problems, one of the parents will often remark, "Just like me when I was young. But back then no one tried to find a cause, and it's too bad, because ..."

Indeed, "back then" no one thought of looking for the reason for such problems in hearing difficulties (unfortunately, they are hardly doing so today, either!) and parents punished or rewarded as the circumstances suggested, and we reached our goals with a lot of work and will power.

The deficiencies we find in children are frequently present in adults also, but the adults I have examined did not complain about the inconveniences they experienced, as I would have expected them to. With perseverance and effort they had managed to overcome their handicap. As they were growing up, the routine of speech and daily reading helped the brain to instantly decode incorrect sound information without error or fatigue. But the concentration this demanded must have made the school years and academic achievement more difficult than it was for others.

A German scientist once devised an experiment that provided a remarkable example of the human capacity to adapt. This doctor wore a pair of glasses which, because of their focal distance, reversed all the images on the retina. He was then operating in a world in which all people and objects were perceived as being upside down, though of course it was only his perception that had changed.

The confusion this caused was quite intense as you might imagine. The researcher nevertheless continued the experiments and, after a few weeks, the cerebral center of vision took charge and corrected the incoming information, and the experimenter was able to function normally, no longer perceiving the world as inverted. When his theory had been proven, he removed the glasses—and without them his adapted vision center once again turned the world upside down, taking another few weeks to return to its normal state.

We can relate this to hearing difficulties. If a child hears "dish" instead of "fish," and "beeper" for "theater," he will by the time he reaches adulthood have organized and set up some kind of automatic coping response. Even if his work calls for some literary skills, no effects of his longtime handicap will be noticed by others, especially when a discreet consultation of the dictionary will allow him to hone his use of language.

A near-complete overcoming of such a hearing handicap is usually the result of constant work and determination, as well as the support and encouragement of the people around him, both at home and at school.

Where some of these factors are lacking, and more of the problem remains, an individual's adaptation to the requirements of society will be accomplished in areas where syntax is not of the greatest importance; a dyslectic can do well in commerce or be a perfect shopkeeper.

IDENTIFIABLE CHARACTERISTICS IN DISTORTIONS

Suppose that someone who has carried over his early hearing problems into adulthood has in spite of them succeeded socially and in the workplace. Is he out of the woods? He still has an imperfect audiogram according to our standards. Are the distortions recorded there only a reminder of past difficulties? No: an experienced eye can discover disturbing information in them.

RELATIVE HYPERACUTE HEARING

The currently accepted way of studying an audiogram is to focus exclusively on the areas located below the ideal line. The "valleys," which reveal a hearing loss, show the way to diagnosis and treatment. No attention is paid to peaks or groups of peaks above the normal line, which indicate the opposite auditory dysfunction, excessively acute hearing. Hyperacute hearing is a source of problems which range well beyond the auditory. It appears that the exaggerated perception of certain frequencies affects specific areas of the brain, triggering abnormal reactions. In some cases, areas elsewhere than in the brain may be affected.

We have found that hyperaudition on specific frequencies always results in the same identifiable problem. This suggests that, although the perception of sound functions to help us control our auditory environment, it might also produce effects in other cerebral areas and in other parts of the body, as we shall discuss shortly. These areas probably vary according to the frequency or group of frequencies

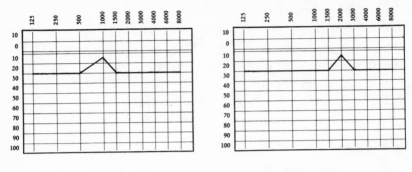

FIGURE 3-1   FIGURE 3-2

perceived by the individual, and react to this abnormal stimulation in a consistent manner.

We discovered that many individuals suffering from allergic disorders such as asthma, hay fever and eczema had hearing peaks in both ears at the frequencies of 1,000, 1,500 and 2,000 Hz. Audiograms for two such individuals are shown in Figures 3-1 and 3-2. That this connection between the allergic problem and hyperacute hearing is significant is indicated by the fact that after appropriate treatment, auditory training which normalized the audiogram and removed the peak or peaks at those frequencies, the patient's symptoms disappeared.

Dr. R. K. Mason of Plymouth College of Technology in England wrote in his article "Asthmatic Sensitivity to High Frequency Sounds":

> One of the characteristics of the asthmatic is a particular sensitivity manifested in his relationship with others. Also, it has been proven that asthmatics are abnormally sensitive to sounds of high frequency—sounds defined between 10 and 30 kHz ... It is possible that high-frequency sounds which appear in speech, sounds which up until now were considered not to mean much, could be useful, especially to children, to communicate emotions. ...

These observations caused us to be particularly alert to

any auditory discrepancy other than hearing loss found in a subject's audiogram.

DEPRESSION

The topic I discuss next may seem surprising, troubling, and for some even nonsensical. Because of this, I feel it necessary to explain in detail the circumstances that brought me to my current level of thinking and understanding.

Around 1970 a sixteen-year-old girl was recommended to me by a psychologist friend. The girl was not responding well to audiogram for a dyslectic problem. We proposed a ten-day course of hearing reeducation, and this was accepted by the psychologist, the girl and her parents. The family lived in another country, so that they had to find a place for their daughter to live during the treatment, and this brought another problem to the fore. The family told us that the daughter was very fragile emotionally, and had already made two attempts at suicide. They felt that it was crucial to find a healthy family with whom she might live in an environment that offered security and affection.

Such a family was found, and the treatment progressed without any problems. At its conclusion the hearing abnormalities had been corrected, as demonstrated by the production of a normal audiogram. The girl returned to her family and her school, promising to get in touch with me in three months to let me know how she was getting on.

After the three months the psychologist who had referred her reported that she was doing well, that all her problems seemed to have cleared up. The psychologist also made an appointment for another patient, a friend of the first girl and asked me, if auditory training turned out to be called for, to make arrangements for her to stay with the family who had lodged her friend. Not only had the first teenager been delighted by her stay with the family, but the new one was as much in need of a supportive environment, having also tried to end her life several times.

We held the consultation and found auditory distortions; treatment proceeded without mishap, producing a normal audiogram; the patient returned home, and, again, I received good news after three months.

Six months later a man of fifty came to me from the south of France for a consultation. His problem was tinnitus, a hearing problem that causes abnormal sounds in the ear, humming, ringing or whistling, and is extremely bothersome for those affected.

This man calmly told me, "These noises are very unpleasant, and if you do not cure me, I shall kill myself. In fact, I have already tried once, and failed, but I guarantee I'll be successful next time."

I spent some time trying to explain to him how to deal with the "crickets" in his head, to reassure him and to guarantee I would do all that was possible. But I was talking to a wall. "Thank you for trying, Doctor," he said. "But I shall commit suicide as soon as I get home if you don't cure me right away!"

I asked more questions, then did a somatic examination and an audiogram.

The audiogram produced a line I had seen before. Naturally, there was a bilateral auditory deficit, which I expected from the interview, but in addition, in the left ear, I saw a familiar graphic image. But of what?

The reader can see by now where I was heading, but at the time I didn't make the connection or even have a clue to what was involved.

Following up this suspicion was very hard work. I went back and studied every audiogram in my files. I finally found six identical pictures, all involving the left ear. And— "of course," you will say!—the audiograms of the two young girls were among them.

My study of the other patients' files revealed that I had noted for each of them episodes of deep depression. The notes were not related to the treatment, but made merely as background information.

Startled by this discovery, I asked my colleagues to let me know of any suicidal patients in their practices so that

I might examine some of them. I was able to do this with several such patients—and in each audiogram the same curve was present for the left ear!

DISCOVERY OF THE 2-8 CURVE

Since then, whenever I do an audiometric examination, I always look to see if the audiogram corresponds, either identically or approximately, to the one which first caught my attention and which showed up in the suicidal patients' audiograms.

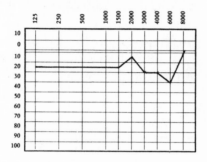

FIGURE 3-3

Figure 3-3 shows the typical curve associated with suicidal tendencies that I noticed when examining my tinnitus patient's audiogram, which triggered my investigation.

The first thing to wonder about is *why* this anomaly, always located on the left side, would coincide with, or perhaps provoke, a suicidal state? The same anomaly on the right corresponds only rarely to a behavioral factor.

The reason is that our cerebral hemispheres do not function symmetrically. As you will recall, the left brain connects to the right ear and deals with speech, action and positive emotion. The right brain is the center of negative emotion linked to mental imagery, and it is the side of the brain which will be affected by any disturbances of the left ear.

In Figure 3-3, typical of a suicidal patient's audiogram, we see hypersensitive hearing at 2,000 Hz, a progressive drop at 3,000, 4,000 and 6,000 Hz, and then an abrupt rise at 8,000 Hz. It is as if the presence of hypersensitivity at the frequencies of 2,000 and 8,000 Hz or the "pulse" produced by these two frequencies were somehow traumatizing to the right brain.

It is not only the peaks on this line that are significant, but the valleys; we see the two areas of hyperacute hearing separated by areas of hearing deficit. A study of the audiograms indicates that the deficits noted at 3,000 and 4,000 Hz are not of importance in this diagnosis. This is fortunate, as a number of people working in excessively noisy environments will show a hearing deficit at 4,000 Hz. It would appear that the determining element is the patient's relative perception of 2,000 and 8,000 Hz in relation to 6,000 Hz—the lowest point on the graph in Figure 3-3.

From now on, for simplicity's sake, we shall refer to this type of audiogram as the *2-8 curve*.

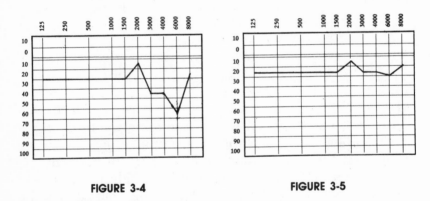

FIGURE 3-4   FIGURE 3-5

Meticulous study of these 2-8 curves and interrogation of our patients has shown without doubt that:

• the deeper the curve between 2,000 and 8,000 Hz (as in Figure 3-4), the more serious is the self-destructive tendency;

• the less pronounced the 2-8 curve, the less serious is this tendency.

The suicidal tendency can in fact remain merely latent, as was the case with the patient whose audiogram is shown in Figure 3-5.

It also appears that the simultaneous presence of a 2-8 curve on the right enhances the destructive potential of a left-ear 2-8 curve.

From the day I first saw that a 2-8 curve on the left represented a suicidal tendency, I found it to be true in all but a few exceptional cases.

All patients who were referred to me by colleagues for suicidal tendencies had a more or less pronounced 2-8 curve on the left. Careful questioning might reveal serious worries about health, family or work, or, on the other hand, a total inability to provide reasons for their wish to kill themselves. The patients in this last category gave answers something like: "No, I have no reason to want to die. I love my husband and my children. We have no financial difficulties or any other serious problem. But at times I can't control myself, and no treatment seems to help."

When patients came to me complaining only of auditory problems, mentioning no other symptoms, and the audiogram showed a 2-8 curve on the left, I felt free to say to them without fear of contradiction, "You forgot to tell me that you sometimes feel suicidal." The confirmation of this comment was always followed by this kind of statement: "Yes, but you don't know what I've had to go through" or "Yes, but I really don't know why."

When a child's audiogram shows the 2-8 curve, the parents always confirm that the child is interested, concerned, even obsessed with death, yet necessarily anxious or afraid. Children's reactions to the concept of death are usually accompanied by some sort of humor meant to show that it is not in the least terrifying to them. For example, the child may look at different models of cars to see if they would make good hearses, or guess what size coffin someone they meet might need, and how many pallbearers it would take to carry him. These instances are typical and by no means exceptional, and show the cast of mind usually encountered when a 2-8 curve exists in the left ear of a child.

The correlation between suicidal tendencies and the 2-8 curve is verified during the course of treatment. When the ten days of auditory training are completed and the new audiogram shows a normal line with the 2-8 curve totally eliminated, the subject resumes normal behavior and suicidal tendencies disappear. This is substantiated by later audiometric examinations and questioning.

Something of the same clinically favorable result is obtained even if only one of the frequencies is flattened, either 2,000 or 8,000 Hz. It is difficult to bring up an auditory curve—that is, to eliminate an area of weak hearing—but comparatively easy to reduce hyperhearing at precise frequencies. In such cases the patient will notice a feeling of psychic well-being, but specify that his depressive or suicidal tendency has not completely disappeared. When this occurs, the treatment has to be stopped for a while, then started again. Luckily, these cases are uncommon.

Sometimes a patient will have a relapse after a few years. Fortunately, this happens only rarely. In one case the patient did not let me know that his suicidal impulses were recurring, but said, "My left ear is acting up." The audiometric examination confirmed the presence of the 2-8 curve.

OTHER CURVES, OTHER CONDITIONS

The discovery of the significance of the 2-8 curve led me to look into possible problems with other frequencies in the neighborhood of 2,000 Hz and their relationship to hyperacute hearing at 8,000 Hz—looking, as it were, for the significance of an "x-8" curve. And indeed this investigation allowed me to relate audiometric disturbances to other behavioral abnormalities.

In particular, I found that, always on the left, simultaneous hypersensitivity at 1,000 and 8,000 Hz (shown in Figure 3-6, we can call this the 1-8 curve) and at 1,500 and 8,000 Hz (the 1.5-8 curve, Figure 3-7) coincide with a depressive state, the depth of which depends on the height of the "hyper" peaks. The 1.5-8 curve generally indicates

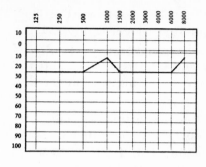

FIGURE 3-6

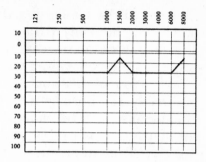

FIGURE 3-7

a more serious condition than the 1-8 curve. In most cases, questioning will reveal patients with a broad range of neuroses (a simple definition of a neurotic is "someone who is not happy with himself"), but who do not ever feel suicidal.

Hyperhearing peaks in both ears at 500 Hz are frequently found in persons with an aggressive personality.

The list of auditory irregularities I have given is far from being complete. Obviously, a rigorous comparison of atypical audiograms with behavior abnormalities will lead to interesting discoveries, especially when testing is done at the intermediate frequencies: 1,100, 1,150, 1,200 Hz, and so on. This research was clearly beyond my scope as a medical doctor, who limited by his clients and work schedule, did not have the time or the number of subjects necessary for in-depth statistical studies.

DIRECT INFLUENCE OF HEARING ON BEHAVIOR

In this chapter I have shown parallels between the auditory state and behavior. The question always asked of me, which has given me a great deal of difficulty, and to which I have given much attention, is:

Does hearing influence behavior or does behavior affect hearing?

This question is an important one, because answering one way or the other leads to completely different therapeutic approaches.

The experiences and observations I have so far presented lead me to the conclusion that the behavior-hearing relationship is not only parallel but one of cause and effect, and, in my opinion, it is the abnormality in hearing that produces the behavioral and emotional problems, and the modification of hearing to correct the abnormalities that is directly responsible for improvements in behavior and emotional state. The elimination of the 1-8 or 2-8 curve on the left always causes the disappearance, often quite quickly, of the depressive or suicidal tendencies, even when all other social or somatic variables have remained the same.

Furthermore, some patients being treated for simple auditory problems reported feeling a negative, unknown and unpleasant state of mind that had not been present earlier. An audiogram showed that their hearing had increased irregularly and that the "traumatizing" frequencies had reached a level higher than that of the other frequencies, temporarily giving the subject a 1-8 or 2-8 curve in the left ear. This artificial state disappeared completely by the end of the twenty sessions.

Obviously this hypothesis would need to be reexamined if we were faced with a subject whose recent audiogram showed no 1-8 or 2-8 curve on the left, but developed one immediately after a psychologically traumatizing experience. This would be an excellent argument for behavior, or experience, modifying hearing; but I have never observed it to happen, and my initial assumption remains my deep conviction.

Do I suggest that all psychoses and neuroses can be cured by otolaryngology? Of course not, any more than all dyslexia and learning disorders can be so cured. I know quite well that each specialist, by his nature, his education, and his experience, is unconsciously biased toward his own therapy, and have tried to be careful not to make this mistake. Nevertheless I feel that we now have a tool that can help educational psychologists faced with the problems of dyslexia and learning disorders, or psychiatrists faced with difficulty in stabilizing behavior by the usual methods. It is not a panacea but a supplement—a very important one—to existing techniques.

Of course, I am well aware of the problems raised by this new technique of diagnosing and treating some cases of the type traditionally dealt with by psychiatry. I also know that my method can be seen as an attack on an entire segment of medicine. I understand fully the questions that will be raised and the difficulties that must be surmounted for the validity of this new process to be verified.

The ideas just presented are not in fact entirely new. Independent of research I undertook in France and elsewhere into the relationship between hearing and dyslexia or hearing and allergies, I came across the work of Dr. Clyde L. Roussey, a child psychologist, and Dr. Ronald Filippi, a psychiatrist at the Menninger Foundation Hospital in Topeka, Kansas. In the early 1960s they presented a report at the International Health Assembly, titled "Detection of Psychiatric Behaviors Through Voice Analysis."

The authors did numerous tests on American and foreign adults, and on 239 children from psychiatric institutions. They taped the subjects' voices and compared the frequency zones recorded to the various behaviors observed, and were able to infer a possibility of diagnosis for specific psychiatric syndromes.

If we know that the sonogram of an individual's voice reflects his hearing, with the vocal cords transmitting the sound perceived and controlled by the ear, we can find an analogy between the results of Dr. Roussey and Dr. Filippi and the theory I have proposed.

Chapter 4

AUTISM

AS I MENTIONED in the introduction, the aspect of my work that has aroused the most attention in the United States is the small portion of it dealing with the baffling "self-imprisonment" of autism. This is partly because of the dramatic cure of this condition in Georgiana Stehli and partly because autism is so little understood and because there is no reliable treatment for it. The case of Georgiana Stehli and of the 47 other autistic patients I have treated indicate that auditory difficulty is often involved in autism and that in such cases auditory retraining can be of help.

What the potential benefit of this approach is to the autistic population in general is only now beginning to be explored, notably in the United States, and we may hope to have solid information on this before too long.

The original edition of this book was written in 1982 and published in France. At that time, responsible medical quarters there did not take a great interest in autism, and even my most persistent attempts to work with specialized centers were fruitless. Therefore my chapter on autism in the earlier version was quite short, in spite of the highly interesting material my work had developed.

Since then, a great deal has happened. For one thing, word-of-mouth contact among parents, both in Europe and in other parts of the world, increased my clientele in this field, providing much more information. For another, I have received a great deal of encouragement and support from specialists in the United States, which looks as if it will lead to great progress in gathering information and developing treatment in this area.

A primary factor is the interest of Bernard Rimland, Ph.D., Director of the Autism Research Institute in San Diego, California in this new approach, completely different from others now in use. Dr. Rimland has asked Steve Edelson, Ph.D., of the Center for the Study of Autism in Newberg, Oregon, to make a controlled pilot study of autistic children.

In addition, several U.S. specialists have come to France during the last few years to be instructed in my methods. And it has become possible, because of the great interest in the field of autism expressed by parents, psychologists, speech therapists and so on, to organize several seminars in the United States at which groups of twenty trainees are trained in applying the methods described in this book, not only in cases of autism but with the other conditions I have discussed.

I look forward to a new era in the study and treatment of autism, made possible by the collation of the results of my consultations with my own patients, of information from seminar graduates concerning those they have treated, and important objective and statistical information from Dr. Edelson's studies. At this point, more than a thousand patients have been treated, and we can look for some clear answers.

That work is very much in progress, and I shall confine my observations in this chapter mainly to the early cases I dealt with, which allowed me to establish my hypothesis on autism.

AUTISM AND COPING WITH IT

The term autism denotes a condition in which patients "refuse" contact, especially verbally, with their environment, and who have other problems of behavior as well, which are sometimes disabling enough to bring about their admission to specialized institutions. It is a disorder of communication and behavior.

Medical research has not yet found any specific treatment for this affliction. For many years there have been experiments with vitamin therapy, with some success. Some medications have been tested—e.g., clonidine and fluoxetine—but the results have not been encouraging or significant enough to lead to definitive conclusions.

The cause of autism is unknown. Research has been conducted into anomalies of the brain, such as hypoplasia (defective development of tissue) of certain portions of the cerebellum, the portion of the brain that transmits sensory information to the motor nerves, or a tumor in some portions of the temporal lobe of the cerebrum, but there is no certitude about this, and it seems possible that there is not one "autism" but several forms, particularly when we consider the different behaviors shown by autistic patients.

Therapies used today have purely functional aims, their goal being to facilitate the inclusion of autistic children in the family environment. The social problems such patients face are harder to solve. There are assistance centers which try to help autistic individuals adjust to the surroundings in which they live.

GEORGIANA: MY FIRST AUTISTIC PATIENT

In 1976, Annabel and Peter Stehli came from the United States to ask if I could treat their 12-year-old daughter, Georgiana. She had been diagnosed as autistic and schizophrenic and was living in a specialized institution in New York called Childville. The Stehlis said they had been advised to consult me because I was known as a specialist in dyslexia and because Dr. William S. Condon of the Boston University School of Medicine had written important articles on the similarity he had found between dyslexia and autism. The most recent, published the previous year in the *Journal of Autism and Childhood Schizophrenia*, was titled "Multiple Response to Sound in Dysfunctional Children."

After reading these articles, I was not yet convinced of the validity of their viewpoint, and explained to the Stehlis that my work was the treatment of hearing anomalies, so that if their daughter had some problems in this area, I would treat them. I told them that I would expect to ameliorate the hearing problems, but could make no promises about the child's behavior, as this was in a totally different area from the learning difficulties I had dealt with by auditory training.

The Stehlis agreed to this, and after several weeks returned with Georgiana. Questioning the parents provided little information bearing on the ear-nose-throat area, except that the girl was afraid of some noises, especially the breaking of ocean waves. A very detailed file from the institution where she had been for the past five years maintained that she suffered from infantile schizophrenia and suicidal tendencies as well as autism; I understood from the Stehlis that the authorities at the institution were vehemently opposed to Georgiana having this treatment or even leaving the premises for long.

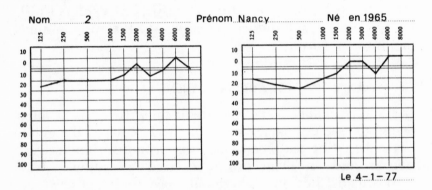

FIGURE 4-1

The audiometric examination was reasonably easy, though the child made some difficulty about accepting the earphones. The audiogram (Figure 4-1) showed some of the usual anomalies associated with dyslexia, principally bilateral distortions. This at least brought her case within the area that I was familiar with, and it was decided to start the treatment immediately.

At first Georgiana refused it, but soon accepted it completely. After a few sessions, she was able to tolerate sounds at an intensity of 100 decibels, which had initially caused her extreme discomfort during a test, though of course sounds of this intensity are not used as part of the treatment.

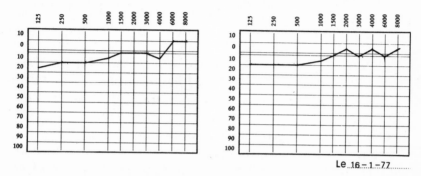

FIGURE 4-2

The improvement of her speech and behavior during the treatment was astonishing, far beyond what either her parents or I had expected. Even a pronounced aggressiveness she temporarily displayed toward her mother was a sign of healing rather than pathology, and she left my office at the end of treatment in effect a different person from the one who had first entered it less than two weeks previously. The audiogram (Figure 4-2) shows the drastic normalization of hearing produced by the treatment.

In less than two months the Stehlis notified me that Georgiana had been integrated into a normal school environment, with no trace of her previous problems. Further reports indicated a complete cure, and by the age of 17 she was involved in a program of advanced studies in design and art and, as I was able to verify in person on a trip to New York in 1982, was an attractive, lively young woman, fluent in English and French, and studying Spanish.

Georgiana's full story is told in her mother's book *The Sound of a Miracle*, which is an excellent picture of the hope and pain involved in any instance of this problem.

FURTHER WORK IN AUTISM

Word of the remarkable result in Georgiana's case spread from parents to parents, and many of them brought their autistic children to us. We noticed that always the parents mentioned one particular auditory abnormality, intolerance of intense sounds. This was usually characterized by a tendency to run away from certain noises while crying or protecting their ears with their hands.

A. G. Gordon in London had already noticed this fact, and wrote in *Medical Hypotheses* for 20 August 1976: "This explains the autistic's inconsistent response to sound. Phonophobia is also another feature, often prominent."

The treatment produced improvement in physiological tolerance to noise, verified by half-hour listening sessions with an intensity of over 60 decibels; and this was often accompanied by improvement in the child's speech and behavior.

None of the other children I saw experienced a complete cure, as Georgiana had, but almost all experienced disappearance of the fear of noise, improvement in behavior, and progressive restoration or improvement in speech; several children who had never spoken developed speech.

There is an obvious objection that will occur to readers of this book, parents, and all categories of specialists interested in autism. The audiogram is the key diagnostic tool, and it is arrived at via the audiometric examination ... which depends upon the accurate responses of the subject. And the very disability which has brought the child to the office is very significantly one of lack of response! How, then, can you obtain an accurate audiogram?

Of course we were faced with this problem from the beginning, and worked hard to find an answer. After having examined and treated many autistic children, and after having verified the information given by our trainees, we have been led to the conclusion that the most important, the main auditory disorder found in autistic patients is *painful hearing*, which, as I said just above, is always mentioned by parents.

It is all too easy to determine which sounds cause pain, and the training device can readily be set to suppress this symptom, even without an audiogram. This allows for some improvement, if not as extensive as might be hoped.

And in some cases it is possible to obtain an audiogram without disturbing the child unduly, and it is then possible to cut the symptomatic hyperhearing peaks as well as dealing with the painful hearing.

None of this is to say that auditory training is *the* treatment of autism. It is only a report on what we have observed and verified: the autistic syndrome is constantly associated with painful hearing. Improvement in behavior occurs when a child's tolerance to intense sound has been achieved.

I feel that it is important to mention that audiometric examination of autistic children sometimes reveals abnormal time responses. Some children answer "too fast." We have observed this same abnormality in Down's syndrome patients, and frequently in schizophrenics. This phenomenon is often confirmed by parents, who say, "We have the feeling he is hearing some sounds even before they are made!"

This and the preceding two chapters have outlined what I have found in my research and in my practice: the relationship of hearing disorders to a great variety of seemingly unrelated problems; broadly, how they are diagnosed; and what can be expected from treatment. I shall now turn to a more detailed discussion of the examinations that determine diagnosis and the treatment that produces such positive results.

Chapter 5

THE AUDIOGRAM

In ORDER to make the accounts of the diagnosis and treatment of dyslexia, learning disabilities, depression and autism understandable, I provided a simplified description of the process of audiometric examination and the production of the audiogram. For those who wish to have a more complete comprehension of this remarkable area of medical science, here is a detailed presentation.

In my experience, the best tool for understanding how an individual truly hears is the pure-tone audiometric examination, which has been in use for many years. Age is the only real limitation on its application: with five-year-olds of reasonable intellectual development it can give valuable indications for a general approach to the problem, and becomes steadily more useful up to the age of ten, at and after which time it is fully applicable.

THE STANDARD AUDIOMETRIC TEST

In this test, the subject sits in a soundproofed room wearing a pair of earphones, after the examiner has checked to make sure there are no obstructions in the external auditory passages. The examiner, either in the same room or in another from which the patient can be viewed through a window, transmits from the audiometer a succession of sounds which vary in both frequency and intensity to each ear in turn.

This test employs the classic audiometer. This device allows us to send to the subject's ears sounds of different frequencies, starting at 125 Hz—that is, 125 vibrations per second—then 250 Hz, 500 Hz and so on up to 8,000 Hz. For each frequency, a control permits the operator to increase or decrease the intensity of the sound, which reaches the subject through headphones.

The first frequency tested is the lowest, 125 Hz, that is, 125 vibrations per second. It is transmitted at first quite faintly, then at greater intensity until the subject indicates that the sound has been heard. This indication can be given in any one of a number of ways: a "yes" or "now," a nod, a gesture of the hand; some types of testing apparatus employ an on-off switch, which is pushed to "on" as soon as the tone is heard. A variation of this links initiation of sound transmittal to the switch, so that the subject controls it.

After the test has established the minimum intensity, measured in decibels, needed for the subject to perceive sound transmitted at 125 Hz, the frequency is increased to 250 Hz, and by stages up to 8,000 Hz, and the lowest decibel level required for perception of each frequency is determined. The maximum decibel level tried in these tests is usually 100 dB.

The results are plotted on a graph called an audiogram, with the frequencies (Hz) being shown on the horizontal axis and the intensity (dB) on the vertical, reading downward from the lowest decibel level at the top.

Each response is entered on the graph, indicating the lowest tone identified for each successive frequency. Connecting these points results in a line, either straight (if all frequencies are heard with the same minimum level of intensity) or irregular (if the minimum intensity levels vary) the area above which represents sounds that the subject cannot hear.

As I mentioned earlier, these tests are performed fully on one ear, and then on the other.

Here is a sample audiogram showing an instance of "normal" hearing that yet shows a modest, not uncommon difference between the two ears.

Figure 5-1 shows that the auditory threshold for the subject's right ear is 10 dB for all frequencies. He can hear no

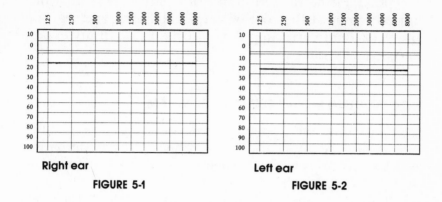

Right ear

FIGURE 5-1

Left ear

FIGURE 5-2

sound transmitted at an intensity of less than 10 dB, but all sounds above that intensity, the more clearly as the intensity increases.

Figure 5-2 shows that the left ear is weaker, since the sound output must reach a level of 15 dB before the subject hears it. Since the subject can hear all frequencies, his hearing will be considered to be 100 percent, and he is not considered to experience any degree of deafness, in spite of the quantitative difference in hearing between the right and left ears.

The audiometric test is followed up with the placement of a vibrator on each mastoid—the bony prominence just behind the outer ear—which can help identify the location of a possible injury. I mention this only in passing, as a full discussion would be complicated and does not bear on the concerns of this book.

The Weber test, on the other hand, is extremely important for our purposes. It employs a vibrator placed in the middle of the forehead, and shows, for each frequency, which ear perceives the sound first. We will discuss this test in detail later in the book.

These tests indicate the nature and scope of hearing loss, and can also assist in the diagnosis and location of an injury. Their most important application in our area of interest is to show which sound frequencies are imperfectly received—for, as we shall discuss next, it is this distorted reception, far more than simple difficulty in hearing, which appears to be at the root of many behavioral and learning problems, and correcting this distortion will, in my experience, usually solve these problems.

HOW TO DO A MORE PRECISE AUDIOGRAM

The pure tone audiogram just discussed gives us a quantitative evaluation of hearing loss, which, greatly simplified, will give us the standard schematic evaluation of deafness at 10 percent hearing loss, 20 percent, 30 percent and so on. This is not the kind of information we look for when doing an audiogram. To explain just what it is we are looking for, we need to look once again at the nature of hearing. In Chapter 2 we discussed extensively the role of hearing in human life from birth or perhaps before, and touched on the bath of sound in which we live. What we must now consider is the condition in which the sound information reaches the brain.

Let us once again use vision as an example. If we take several individuals who have perfect vision and give them, in strictly identical lighting conditions, a group of objects, pictures and printed texts, they will all be able to describe perfectly what they see in terms they can all understand. They will all perceive identical objects identically, which is to say correctly.

If we replace several of these subjects with people suffering from myopia, astigmatism, daltonism or some other uncorrected optical condition, the people involved would see things differently, to nobody's surprise. Complex tests are not needed to verify the evident fact that each person perceives visual material differently. With perfect vision, we know that people see things identically; with defective vision, we know just as well that they see them differently.

In auditory domain, things are different. Who can tell what sound one person perceives or how he perceives it? How can we relate one person's perception of a specific sound to another's of that same sound? Nothing and no one can give that information because of the inherent ephemeral nature of sound.

What then can we do if we suspect the existence of an auditory abnormality other than deafness—an abnormality that might cause an alteration in the reception of external sound?

Let us look at an audiometric examination designed to help us find some answers and which will give us a great deal of information—the information, in fact, which has been touched on in previous chapters without the full explanation of how it was arrived at.

We said in Chapter 1 that the sound spectrum humans perceive is spread between the frequencies of 15 Hz and 20,000 Hz, the actual range varying with the individual. We limit our examination to the area between 125 Hz and 8,000 Hz, which corresponds to the range of frequencies of conversation and sounds encountered in everyday life. We have noticed that the afflictions we treat are related to auditory problems located within this range.

FACTORS IN TESTING

1. The room

Of course, the examination room must be soundproofed in order to avoid having the subject's ear disturbed by noise coming from the outside. However, we have noticed that the soundproofing cannot be absolute, and there is a good psycho-physiological reason for this: the subject, already a little anxious because of the test, can be made even more so by an abnormal sound environment. For one thing, the voice of the operator will be heard in a manner other than normal because of the absence of all ordinary noises. For another, the sound stimulus from the equipment will be received by the auditory system in an abnormally precise context, giving us no clue about how it would be perceived by the subject under ordinary conditions—and that is precisely what we are trying to find out!

When tests have been given in an absolutely sound-proofed area, the subject has perceived the sounds produced by his own body: intestinal rumbling, heartbeat, inner-ear blood circulation. His own voice seemed strange and foreign to him; he felt uneasy. It is evident that an audiometric examination given under these conditions will not give us the information we want.

A little ambient sound should "leak" in to the examination room, but it should not be located where street sounds, music or noise from other rooms can be heard.

2. The audiometer

It must in all cases include a complex system of handles which allows the detection of voluntary or involuntary errors made by the subject. These are necessary to permit correction of such errors and, as we shall see later, to study the quality of the answers.

3. Subjects' responses

Traditional methods of response are a switch to give a sound or light signal, nods or hand gestures indicating "yes (I hear the sound)" or "no (I've stopped hearing it)," and too-long sentences. We have stopped using any of them, as they generate errors. Since they are still in wide use, I will take a moment to explain why we do not employ them.

Switch. When involved with an advanced examination, the operator has a tendency to send sound messages to the subject at a very rapid speed; and it is possible for the subject to press or release the switch at the wrong time without the operator noticing the error.

Finger signals. We frequently saw subjects who, when very absorbed in the task of listening to a barely audible sound, would raise an index finger when the sound had just stopped. Faced with our surprise, they would say, "Wait, I am trying to find out if I am hearing anything." Had we just noted this gesture as a positive answer, our records would have been wrong and the subject credited with some very odd responses.

Nods. I can affirm that the up-and-down "yes" and the side-to-side "no" are constant sources of confusion. The subject usually continues his vertical nod of assent while

66

the intensity of the emitted sound diminishes, and right past the actual cessation of the sound.

I believe that it is impossible to get a precise audiogram with these flawed methods. I know many audiologists will disagree with me, but the problems with these widely used techniques seem to me to explain the fact that two audiograms done on the same person but given by two different operators are rarely superimposable, and can even present some strong disparities. Still, the result of these disparities is minimal when we are only looking for a global evaluation of the ear.

When doing an audiogram, I ask the subject—to be frank, I insist—to answer orally with a "yes" or "no" or "I don't know." These responses are unambiguous, and can be verified immediately if there is any doubt. At the outset the subject understands that he must notify the examiner by saying "yes" as soon as he hears a sound and "no" at the disappearance of the sound.

4. The operator

It is absolutely necessary that the person administering the test be able to evaluate the subject psychologically if he is to recognize how the person reacts to sound.

First of all, he must explain patiently and clearly what the examination consists of. He must be reassuring, and, when working with children, smile often, so that they will feel as if they are taking part in a game rather than experiencing the stress of a test. Or he may need to reassure an adult subject so as to make him feel less anxious about the result. It is, in fact, surprising to see how often the subjects, regardless of their age, worry to the point of traumatization about the test.

When the operator notices that an error has occurred, he must inform the subject and explain carefully that he is able to detect errors. If these errors persist, the operator must make a record of the observed abnormalities, in addition to the information noted in the audiogram. We shall touch on this a little later.

5. The observer

We encourage the presence of a family member, a parent or spouse. We ask such a person to remain for the whole examination, from the initial explanation to the subject, right through to the end. This is by far the best way for those close to the person being tested to understand what is involved in his or her condition.

The observer is required to maintain absolute silence and immobility, but the operator may indicate by finger gestures any obvious abnormality, qualitative or quantitative, in the subject's responses. The observer is thus prepared to understand the later explanation of the audiogram's results, while to the subject it is often only a rather uninformative diagram.

When a parent is present at an examination, he can understand just why his child needs treatment; and with adult subjects, having a family member present often helps the whole family accept the need for treatment. For example, the subject's condition might require surgery or the wearing of a hearing aid, or long-term medical treatment, even treatment that does not show immediate results, or eventual retraining of the ear. Above all, having a representative at the examination can lead to the family understanding that they must adapt their speech patterns and habits to the subject's hearing capacity.

Another advantage of having an observer at the examination is that the family can see more clearly what improvements come with treatment.

ABNORMALITIES TO BE LOOKED FOR

In Chapter 2 I mentioned eight abnormalities commonly encountered in testing and discussed them in relationship to children's hearing problems, saying that I would go into them in greater detail later on; and now is the time for that.

1. Problems in response timing

As mentioned, the normal interval between a sound stimulus and the response to it is about a second, but it can be longer—or, surprisingly, shorter.

a) Slow responses. Especially with children, we can notice a reaction time of two, three, four, even five seconds. When we notice such a slow reaction, we ask the child if he has understood what is expected, and he will almost always indicate that he does: a "yes" as soon as a sound is heard, and a "no" when it stops. And when the examination continues, the slow response time persists.

Where, anatomically and physiologically, in the transmission-response circuit the delay is located is certainly a knotty question. It is not, however, one that is of immediate concern in this situation. We are interested only in the amount of time the response to the sound stimulus takes and not in the area causing the delay. The delay becomes a greater hindrance when, instead of a single sound, we give the subject some complex sentences composed of a multitude of sound groups, or phonemes.

b) Fast responses. We do not include in this category answers given in a rush by a child eager to be finished with the examination, by a highly impulsive child, or by one eager to impress. Such answers are characterized by the constant presence of errors, and the matter is one of the psychoneurotic aspects of response, to be commented on later.

But we do need to pay special attention to responses that are practically instantaneous, and whose rapidity seems almost to anticipate the stimulus. The "yes" and "no" happen at the precise moment that the sound is sent or cut, whatever precautions the operator takes to conceal any movement that might provide a clue to what is about to happen.

This almost nonexistent response time is always tied to identical clinical symptoms. It is interesting to notice that these subjects often seem almost unconcerned over the examination. They seem distracted, look around, play with their fingers, but never make an error, no matter what the variety of traps set for them.

c) Retention. This is what happens when a subject gives his response to the sound at the moment of its emission, but his response to the cut-off of the sound is not nearly as precise. This can make it difficult to get an absolutely accurate audiogram.

The subject never responds to the interruption of the sound with a precise "no," as called for. Instead, he responds with a sentence and a doubt: "I don't know if it's your machine or if I still have the sound in my ear from before." The same situation is repeated with the transmission of other sounds. This abnormality, independent of all physiological effect, is to be found, audiologists have observed, among intellectuals who try to reason out their impressions rather than respond with the simple monosyllables called for.

2. Errors

Wrong answers can make audiometric examinations complex and exacting for the operator and probably for the subject as well, since they demand extra attention on the part of both and increase the length of time the test takes.

The errors are easily identified by cross-checking the results obtained during the first systematic examination and then doing random retakes. Random retakes will not permit the subject to answer in any manner he can anticipate, responding, for example, "yes" to the first two questions and "no" to a third.

When several mistakes are made, it is necessary to explain once more to the subject what is expected of him and to show him the types of mistake he made. If the answers continue to be incorrect, this must be noted.

3. Fatigue

Usually the audiogram is done from beginning to end in a standardized manner. The response time, normal, fast or slow, remains the same from beginning to end. Sometimes, during the examination, the rhythm slows down progressively, usually accompanied by a diminution of tonality in the voiced response—it becomes atonal—and an increase in the number of errors. Everything happens as if the subject became tired of listening, or tired of making the effort to answer correctly.

Sometimes, if an effort is not made to stimulate him, the audiometric examination may end with the subject in a deep sleep.

4. Painful hearing

In normal hearing, whatever the frequency being tested, as the sound intensity is progressively increased, say from 20 dB to 110 dB, the maximum reached with ordinary audiometers, the subject will respond by saying, "It is louder and louder." At around 100 dB, he will give the appropriate response, "It is very loud." If, with the proper equipment, 130 dB is reached, the subject will start to make faces, and at 140 dB will make gestures indicating that he is in pain.

With other subjects the complaint of loudness can be made soon as 40 dB is reached, generally accompanied by a frown. An additional 5 dB of intensity will often bring the subject to say, "You're hurting me!" If we increase the intensity further, the subject will whip off the earphones. The elasticity, the normal range of hearing tolerance, instead of going beyond the 100 dB level, is reduced to about 50 dB, a good deal less in certain cases. It is also possible for a subject to begin hearing sound only when an intensity of 60 dB has been reached, and for the sound to become intolerable to him at 80 dB.

This intolerance is usually associated with the higher sound frequencies, and typically the subjects show an auditory deficit at these same frequencies. Sometimes individuals with audiograms showing no such deficit display this intolerance.

An analogy is the situation of an individual who is suffering from limited mobility of the elbow. A normal elbow can bend or stretch over a range of about 130 degrees, from straight out to folded. After a break, mobility can be reduced to as little as 40 degrees. In some cases this is the result of the mechanical interference of bone calcification; in others, there is accompanying pain that increases with the extent of the attempted flexion. There are also cases in which the elbow can move through its full normal range, but only with severe pain. X-rays will show no abnormality, but the elbow is limited in its ability to function. This is comparable to the intolerance some people experience to various levels of sound.

5. Lack of selectivity

After verifying that the subject understands the difference between high-pitched and low-pitched sounds, and after testing him several times at the extreme frequencies, 125 Hz and 8,000 Hz, we have him listen, with an average intensity of 50 dB, to a succession of sounds of progressively descending frequency. We start at the highest, 8,000 Hz, then go to 6,000 and so on down to 125 again; and then back up to 8,000 Hz.

At each step the subject is asked if the sound is higher or lower than the preceding one. Often the answers given are accurate, but sometimes they are incredibly off. A subject may claim that 6,000 Hz is a higher tone than 8,000 Hz, but then report perfectly accurately the lowering of tones at 4,000, 3,000 and so on.

We often find a range of wrong answers spread over a large range of frequencies, which can extend from 8,000 to 1,000 Hz. A subject will say, "Higher ... higher again" to each lowering of the tone, and then stay silent when a 500 Hz tone is transmitted immediately after one of 1,000 Hz. Why? Because, he claims, "it is the same sound"!

Another person may manifest "bands" of errors. For example, wrong answers may prevail for the frequencies between 8,000 and 4,000 Hz; answers between 4,000 and 2,000 Hz will be accurate; errors again between 2,000 and 1,000; and at last correct answers from 1,000 to 125 Hz.

On the return trip up to 8,000 Hz, we generally find mistakes in the same areas in which they appeared on the descent.

We might well wonder if the subject has lost track of what he is supposed to be doing, or has given up on the test and is just saying whatever comes into his mind! That is not the answer, though, since the same test, given several times over a period of some days, shows the same errors at the same frequencies. These test results show that the subject truly hears what he says he does, however far that is from what was actually transmitted through the earphones.

All this concerns the testing of one ear only, let us say the right one. When we go to the left ear, the surprises are not over. The left ear may exhibit the same abnormalities as the right; or we might notice a completely different set of errors, even a reversal, with the tones perceived as rising in one ear being heard as descending in the other. Or testing the left ear may give us perfectly correct responses. If that happens, it is common for the subject to volunteer such a comment as: "Oh, you know, I don't hear the same in both ears!"

6. Auditory distortions

Perfect hearing is shown on an audiogram by a perfectly horizontal line. This indicates that the subject hears sound in all frequencies with the same intensity, if the examiner has transmitted at a constant level.

To illustrate, suppose that we hit all the keys of a piano, from left to right, with the same force. We will produce sounds of ascending frequency but the same intensity, and should be able to hear them at the same level of intensity: the C should not seem louder than E flat an octave higher or than F sharp an octave lower.

Figure 5-3 shows an example of perfect hearing. The

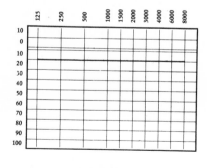

FIGURE 5-3

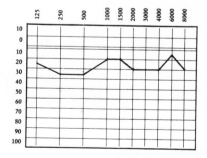

FIGURE 5-4

subject begins to hear sounds starting with an intensity of 10 dB. If he is next sent the sounds at an intensity of 50 dB, he will report the tone changes but specify that the intensity remains level.

In Figure 5-4 we see an irregular line, which indicates an excellent reception of frequencies at 1,000, 1,500 and 6,000 Hz, in contrast with less satisfactory reception at 250, 500, 2,000, 3,000, 4,000 and 8,000 Hz. This means that the first frequencies are perceived at a sound level less intense than those of the other six.

If for one ear that produced this audiogram a succession of sounds is produced with a constant intensity of 10 dB, the answers will be "no" for all frequencies other than 1,000, 1,500 and 6,000 Hz. If the decibel level is increased to 40 dB, then the subject will respond "yes" each time, but he will tell you that he hears 1,000, 1,500 and 6,000 Hz much louder than the other frequencies.

You can readily imagine the variety of audiograms that can be obtained for each ear with the ten frequencies fully tested. Later on, we will look at the wealth of information the audiologist can obtain by studying these diagrams.

The importance we attach to this type of abnormality explains in part my insistence on the necessity for a precise audiometric examination. All differences in decibel level between two neighboring frequencies must be noted, even if such differences are minimal, because they strongly affect diagnosis.

7. Auditory laterality

Now we return to the Weber test, a standard one; but we shall require of it something more than usual. Different frequencies, from 1,500 to 4,000 Hz, are applied to the frontal bone, directly on the midline of the skull, and the subject indicates from what direction the frequency seems to come. The sound may be reported as coming from the right, from the left, from the center, from behind, even "from everywhere." We discussed the nature of laterality and the consequences of dyslaterality in Chapter 2, and noted there that the Weber test, used in this manner, allows us to locate the areas in which this problem arises.

8. *Psychoneurotic aspects of responses*

This area is particularly interesting when a child is tested. The manner of response often gives a clear idea of the subject's usual behavior, which is confirmed by the parent or other observer who knows the child. There are several types of behavior which we have observed to recur in testing.

There are those children who are completely absorbed in the examination. They enjoy wearing the earphone apparatus like a spaceman's helmet, and treat the examination as a game they are participating in, which we encourage them to do from the beginning, and relish the congratulations they receive for correct answers. All these factors result in such children applying themselves very carefully and diligently to the test.

Another category consists of "shrewd" children who, as soon as an error is brought to their attention, no longer try to answer accurately, but try only to outwit the operator. They watch the operator's hands for clues rather than listening for the sound; in effect, they try to short-circuit the examination process. The parents usually confirm that this is how such children normally behave. They try to find all possible shortcuts in order to avoid unpleasant tasks, even though, as in mountain climbing, these shortcuts sometimes show themselves to be more difficult than the prescribed route. Dealing with a subject like this can be enormously tiring for the operator who is trying to get an accurate audiogram.

Others are just not interested in the examination. They seem to answer virtually at random. They do not seem to care about the congratulations they receive for good answers or about the gentle reprimands for obvious fantasies. They play with their fingers or with the earphone cord, they swing their legs, they glance restlessly at their parents, the operator, the controls on the audiometer. We constantly have to remind them of the examination in progress, and the parents almost always confirm that this is the kind of thing that happens at school and at home.

Others want to do too much, and challenge you, for example saying "Oh, yes, sir, I am sure I heard something" when no sound whatever was transmitted. They show off during the examination as they do in outside life.

These are just a sample of the personalities one might come across; and, however engaging or demanding they are, their varied behavior is highly informative about their basic personality.

Chapter 6

TREATMENT

THERE ARE many auditory dysfunctions to which auditory training can usefully be applied, but neither it nor any other treatment offers a certain cure for all the problems we have discussed. Before we look into auditory training, we should touch on the traditional methods of dealing with hearing problems.

STANDARD TREATMENTS

In this area, as in every medical area, the first thing necessary is to ask careful questions, then do a thorough medical examination, so as to obtain an accurate diagnosis of any existing physiological problem. Such a diagnosis may well result in directing a patient toward one of the traditional solutions such as medication, surgery, thermal treatment or a hearing aid.

But if none of these is useful, for instance because the transmission blockage in the eardrum is not sufficient to justify remedial steps, or because abnormalities such as those we have examined—slowness in response, painful hearing, auditory distortions and so on—do not respond to any traditional treatment, what is to be done?

In my practice, I tried to avoid a narrow approach. My training and the requirements of my profession, and the eventual development of my interest in the linkage between hearing and behavior, obliged me to develop several areas of expertise, to become an "omni-practitioner" in the largest medical-surgical sense. Different situations put me in contact with various medical and paramedical disciplines, as well with different cultural backgrounds. Through this exposure I came to realize that medical truth has several facets, and that there is no one true road to health.

I have, however, found that auditory training is often an excellent route, and have followed it to achieve the results described in earlier chapters.

RETRAINING THE AUDITORY SYSTEM

1. Fundamentals

It is well known that a patient with a type of polio resulting in a functional deficiency of a limb (through muscular atrophy resulting from nerve injury) has a good chance of recovering partial or total mobility of the limb by undergoing appropriate physiotherapeutic treatment. There are many examples of athletes who, struck in childhood by a viral attack and a dire prognosis, overcame their affliction through will power and specialized training. They achieved not merely functional rehabilitation but near-superhuman results of a kind which at the onset of their illness would have seemed inconceivable.

This is not to suggest that physical therapy revives a dead muscle, not at all; no one believes that. What actually happens is that neighboring muscles and muscular fibers remaining in the affected area increase their potential, just as a healthy nervous system compensates for a destroyed nerve.

Cannot what takes place in the muscular and nervous systems be possible elsewhere? About fifty years ago there was some interesting work in visual retraining done by William Bates in England, which appeared to have some encouraging results. It has been neglected lately, though some recent research has been reported from Japan. *Whatever the merits of the approach eventually prove to be, it does appear that functional deficiencies in the eye can in some measure be compensated for by retraining.* If this is so for the eye, why not for the ear?

In the last several years a number of sound processing centers have opened in Europe and in the United States.

These establishments attempt to cure hearing problems with a variety of techniques, ranging from simply listening to tapes of music, selected according to the operator's subjective assessment of the patient, to much more sophisticated methods using filtered sounds supposedly reproducing the intrauterine hearing of the fetus. These approaches, whatever their worth, bear only a distant resemblance to the auditory retraining concept, based upon the most precise audiographic testing of the patient.

In discussing intolerance to certain frequencies in the previous chapter, I touched on an analogy with an injured elbow and the limitations this imposes. Let me now take this a step further and move on to the treatment for the elbow and its similarity to auditory retraining.

After medical treatment and the use and removal of a cast, the patient has a stiff elbow, with movement and flexibility limited to an arc of 30 degrees, accompanied by pain and possible muscular weakness.

This patient might be sent to one practitioner who makes him exercise the arm with flexions and extensions over an arc of less than 30 degrees. This will be quite comfortable to the patient, and almost completely worthless. Or he might be sent to a more forceful one, who physically forces the articulation to increase to 60 or 70 degrees. Result: severe pain and very likely an aggravation of the injury.

What usually happens, luckily, is that the patient is sent to a physical therapist who knows his job. The therapist matches his efforts to the problems and the reactions of the patient, so that the angle of articulation is gradually increased and the therapist exercises the muscles in a progressive manner, not traumatizingly.

The result is that, after a reasonable number of sessions, the limb will have recovered its mobility and be pain-free, perhaps completely, but at least to the extent of showing a clear improvement.

I have made it my rule to follow to the best of my ability this kind of purely mechanical orientation in auditory retraining.

You may say that the problem is not the same. Flexing an elbow is by no means as complex as the synergistic process necessary to interpret sound, from its initial introduction at the outer ear to its microsecond-long journey along a tortuous pathway to the relevant parts of the brain; and in addition to the inherent complexity of transmission, obstacles may interfere with it at many different points along the way.

That is true, but remember the German researcher who brought about a complete reversal of visual perception? This is an incredibly complex neurological process, but the method used was direct and simple—one might almost say crude—an inverting lens. It is my contention that hearing reeducation is no more complicated than this.

In order to restore the elbow's mobility, the physical therapist must make it perform movements of flexion, of extension, of external and internal rotation, progressively forcing the action without traumatizing the elbow. Similarly, it is necessary to bring to the ear sounds which will make it work, sounds which are alternately stronger, softer, higher, lower, originating from the left and from the right. This must be done with a bearable, nonaggressive but still therapeutic intensity. It must also have an appropriate rhythm; alternating the sounds too quickly or too slowly would diminish the effectiveness of the training.

The audiogram of each subject determines the adjustment of the reeducating transmitter. Obtaining an audiogram is at best a taxing process for the operator, and for the subject, who must at times discriminate between tones only 5 dB apart in intensity. The process is, naturally, more difficult with children; and when the children are nonverbal or have 30-second attention spans (with a minimum of 20 minutes being required), there is no chance of getting a worthwhile audiogram. This is why we were able to get audiograms for only 12 of the 48 autistic children we tested.

2. *Technique*

The sound used in auditory retraining is produced by an electronic device especially built to my specifications after a good deal of clinical trial-and-error research.

The first problem we were faced with was the source of the sound the instrument was to transmit. A traditional approach was to use the subject's own voice, modified as needed and then sent to him through the earphones. The inconveniences of this technique soon became apparent. It was difficult to obtain a good thirty-minute recording of the subject's voice to use. It was difficult to record at a sufficient and constant intensity, with acceptable tonal quality and speech rhythm. The subject would tire quickly, and the number of recording sessions required was excessive.

We then used commercial records, and, later on, more and more elaborate audiotapes. Later still, the tapes were filtered to remove those frequencies which the audiogram indicated were injurious.

Transforming these tapes for therapeutic use presented enormous technical problems; but things are a great deal easier now. Thanks to the progress of electronics and the skill of the technician who perfected our instruments, the latest model can take a standard music tape and filter the required sounds as well as produce the desired sound modulations. Although the auditory problems treated are located between 125 Hz and 8,000 Hz, our instrument provides frequencies from 30 Hz to 15,000 Hz to provide a more dynamic treatment.

With the early auditory retraining machines, we had to use tapes that had been prepared from selected music tapes and records, with certain frequencies filtered. Over the years we have developed a new system, known as the Ears Education and Retraining System (E.E.R.S.); it makes use of many different sound sources—LP records, compact discs, cassettes—making available a substantial quantity and variety of intensities. The last pattern, using the newest discoveries of electronic science, is the *kinetron*.

The system alternates low and high sounds in an irregular pattern, so that the patient does not become accustomed to the rhythm. Filters attenuate the traumatizing frequencies, while the intensity is determined by the original source. As the sounds are produced, they are modified; higher, lower, louder, softer, filtered, unfiltered. They are controlled in such a way that they cannot affect the patient traumatically, no matter what hearing problem he presents.

Guided by both the initial audiogram and that taken at midpoint in the treatment, the operator adjusts the instrument—the latest version is known as the Kinetron—to alter frequencies, intensities and lateralization of the sounds.

The auditory treatment consists of 20 half-hour sessions of retraining. Though the session length may appear short, experience has shown that it is sufficient, and that a longer session would be unnecessary and perhaps counterproductive. If no positive result is observed after 10 hours of treatment, it usually appears that the technique is of no use in that case, and that extending the sessions would not help.

All this seems quite complicated; why not, you may ask, just listen to some music at home?

The problem and its remedy are more complex than that. If we look again at the example of the elbow, a normal elbow can make all sorts of movements: flexion, extension, rotation. It can be exercised vigorously and thus be made stronger. But an injured elbow is restricted in movement, and any uncontrolled effort (such as that made by our forceful second practitioner) will not help the condition but aggravate it.

The same is true of hearing. A normal ear can withstand fairly loud noise, although after a while repeated traumatizing sounds will affect it, probably first at 4,000 Hz and then at the frequencies close by. An ear manifesting a hearing problem as indicated by an abnormal audiogram will have much less resistance to certain frequencies. An unlimited absorption of decibels can aggravate the situation by trying to "over-reeducate" the abnormal frequencies the person already hears. At the same time this sound tires the ear in areas where frequencies were not heard as well, which can also increase the initial distortions.

ASPECTS OF THE TREATMENT

The treatment consists of three phases.

1. Auditory diagnosis and identification of the type of retraining needed, entailing:

   a) a thorough consultation with the patient and his family, including looking into hereditary aspects and personal history; and
   b) an ENT examination and initial audiogram.

2. Observation of the patient's behavior and reactions during the 10 days of treatment; a monitoring audiogram is done halfway through the treatment, after the tenth session.

3. Evaluation of the results:
   a) a final audiogram and evaluation of the patient's auditory capacity is done after the 20 sessions;
   b) behavior changes are evaluated after three months.

The two aspects of the first phase have been discussed in the preceding chapters, as was the first part of the last phase. In this connection I should point out that the evaluation of results mentioned refers only to the area of hearing presented by the change in the audiogram. I shall discuss the second phase and the three-month evaluation in the next sections.

BEHAVIOR DURING THE 20 SESSIONS

Early in my work I was intrigued by remarks often made by the parents and the children we saw, though I did not attach much significance to them. These remarks covered many areas and seemed to have nothing much in common. Here, in no particular order, are the remarks made most frequently:

- My child is delighted to come and listen to some music.
- He refuses to come to you.
- Yesterday he started to sing in the street at the top of his voice.
- He complained of a stomachache and threw up his lunch.
- She eats twice as much as before.
- He complains of headaches.
- His headaches have disappeared.
- She asked that we buy her some books, something that has never happened before.
- He is more affectionate.
- She had an incredibly aggressive tantrum.
- He was horribly rude.

All this abnormal behavior was blamed, as much by the families as by me, on the change of routine: living in a hotel; interruption of school and a vacation taken at an unusual time; having to come to the doctor's office twice a day at specific times; and a modification of family relationships.

In short, there was a whole spectrum of new conditions, pleasant or not, to which the children appeared to react in accordance with their personalities, and also according to the weather. Annecy is a wonderful city when the weather is nice, and the young people delight in the lake and the mountain. Naturally, they are less delighted at the idea of stopping short at four o'clock sharp to be at the doctor's by 4:30. This in itself did not seem to create any noticeable problem.

However, a certain sameness developed in conversations with parents bringing their children in for their appointments, and this particular exchange seemed to happen over and over again:

"Good morning, Madame, and how is Jean-François today?"

"Well . . . fine, Doctor, but he threw a real tantrum when we had to get him out of the pool to come to see you."

"Oh, this isn't so bad—we'll get through the 'torture'

quickly and he can get back to having fun." A pat on the cheek for Jean-François, and a chocolate bar if that seemed called for, and the session would go on, with everything back in order.

Adult subjects also expressed some negative feelings, but these were more personal and focused on the tapes used in the sessions. "Yesterday I was doing fairly well, but you made me listen to some Tchaikovsky! That ruined the day, and I went to bed without dinner."

Poor old Tchaikovsky! But it didn't seem to be his fault, especially with another patient telling me just as strongly, "At last an interesting half hour! That 'Nutcracker' is sublime!"

The two critics illustrate the swings from negative to super-positive responses I began to notice after I had been involved in the treatment for some time. The children could experience moments of incredible joy as well as moments of feeling the blues, discouragement or aggression. This elation also interfered with the routine of administering the test, and required a few calming words from me before we could proceed.

After I had worked with a large number of patients and had heard such remarks and observed such responses many, many times, I realized that it all made sense, and that there was a deep and unique reason for this phenomenon of strong emotional reaction, positive and negative, to the treatment.

It was the audiogram administered after the tenth session that gave me a clue. (After the tenth session, halfway through the retraining, we always do an audiogram to verify the tuning of the retraining instrument, which was based on the initial audiogram; the new one verifies any satisfactory results obtained.) We found that the more improvement shown by the tenth-session audiogram, the stronger was the intensity of the patient's reaction.

As soon as I realized this I began to note each reaction systematically, recording the date on which it appeared and its duration. A curve based on this data established that the greatest number of reactions took place around the seventh session and that their rate decreased in a shallow curve toward the end of the treatment.

My conversations with my patients and their parents changed. Small talk gave way to precise questions: What reactions were noticed? After which session? How many hours or days did they last? The information I got from this allowed me to make some modifications in the treatment.

The reaction noticed most often was a fatigue of variable intensity and duration. In some extreme cases a child would spend several hours asleep for each day of the treatment. Others simply mentioned excessive fatigue, or a sudden feeling of sleepiness during the middle of the day.

The second group of reactions has no single identifying characteristic, but includes all the little abnormalities mentioned earlier: depression, aggression, elation, joy, discouragement. I feel that it is necessary to mention aggressiveness, because this feeling occurs quite often, and because of the conclusions I have drawn concerning it. The aggressive reaction can sometimes appear suddenly and violently, in a manifestation that neither the patient nor the family expects. And when that happens, there is no apparent external reason for it. It is usually a matter of words or obstructive behavior, but is sometimes expressed physically, e.g., with punches and kicks, directed primarily at the mother. This symptom usually disappears after a day, though it can sometimes last longer.

Aside from the characteristic chronology—the quick beginning and fairly quick resolution of the reaction—I noticed other things that helped in dealing with the problem. Specifically:

• The aggressive crisis is always minimized, if not completely forgotten, by the patient. He will listen to the account of his behavior with surprise or indifference, and say, "Well, that's normal."
• The quicker and the more violent the physical reaction, the better the audiometric results are; and, later on, im-

provements in school work will be correspondingly satisfactory.

• It is important not to use physical restraint; we have had to use medication sometimes, but always mild.

Patients' reactions during treatment vary quite a lot. I am giving the aggressive factor attention here because of its spectacular aspect, and because it might worry people who are not prepared for it. I want to advise parents to be aware that a kind of "mental storm" may take place. Although it may be violent, it is always beneficial, and seems to be part of the process of the cure. Why this should be so is still a mystery.

With adults—typically, those suffering from suicidal depression—the initial reaction is an increasing tendency toward irritability, followed by progressive improvement. The critical time is much longer than it is for a child, and lasts for several days.

It is important for the patient to understand thoroughly how the treatment will progress. In particular, he must absorb the fact that treatment is a matter of stabilizing a defective hearing system, and that psychotherapy is in no way involved. He should experience no anxiety if he understands that any adverse reaction is physiologically based and short-lived.

For adults who have the same type of reactions as children, we advise great caution in the use of medications.

From the outset, patients are now warned in detail of the unpleasant secondary reactions that might occur and told of the positive role they play in the treatment. However, to avoid disturbing them in case the effects are in fact not apparent, we also let them know that:

• Reactions sometimes appear as hypersensibility or as an extreme expression of affection.
• The absence of a reaction is not to be taken as indicating failure of the treatment; perhaps a reaction may simply not occur, or it is so short as not to be noticed, or it

might take place without any witnesses, such as during the night as the patient is dreaming.

My documentation of the different reactions, some quite traumatizing, would fill a large book, but I shall limit myself here to three typical cases.

Some years ago a six-year-old boy, the youngest of five children, was brought to us by his mother from the small country village where they lived. The teacher had told the parents, "Your child is absolutely not keeping up with the class; he is always distracted and looks away when we speak to him, and I wonder if he hears properly. You should take him to a hearing specialist."

The results of the consultation showed problems in the middle ear, a light inflammation, and some pronounced auditory distortions; retraining seemed clearly necessary. I tried to explain the process to the mother, who put me at ease immediately: "After all, Doctor, we understand nothing and we trust you. Treat him as you see fit."

To my warning of possible reactions, she said, "We have plenty of work on the farm with the animals and five kids, and we don't have any time to notice bad behavior."

On the morning of the fifth day, after eight sessions, the mother brought her son in and gave us the details of the preceding day, which were certainly noticeable.

At noon the family sat down to eat ... without the youngest. They called him once, twice, with no response. The father got angry, went out and found the boy playing with the chickens, and asked him if he had not heard him call. The child answered that he had, and could not see why it was always the father who decided when they should eat. This drew a quick slap from the father, and the child ran away; the family went after him, but the child eluded them.

An hour later the village priest brought him back, holding him by the ear. The child had met him on the road, he said, jumped onto him, clawing at his clothes, and had cursed him like a sailor. The mother remembered my warnings, and intervened to prevent the spanking which was clearly the next item on the agenda. The child went to bed voluntarily, saying that "it was enough."

In my office, the child listened absentmindedly to the story as if it had nothing to do with him.

This incident was the only one, and lasted about an hour. The father never did understand what had taken place, which was a sudden catharsis of all the feelings he had against his family and, presumably, the church.

At about the same time, an upper-class woman from Geneva brought in her twelve-year-old daughter, who was dyslexic. The questions and examinations went ahead with no problems. Our hearing evaluation and recommendation for treatment in Annecy were well accepted by the mother, who had already arranged to have the child taken care of by friends of the family. The mother interrupted our warnings of possible behavior reactions, including the use of bad language, with a condescending smile: "Doctor, this would surprise me greatly. In our family, thank God, the children have had a proper upbringing, and we never have any problem of this sort."

The following Monday morning, my secretary told me that the mother was on the telephone, and not at all happy. I took the call.

"Doctor, this is shameful! I should have known about you and the people my daughter stayed with! It's terrible! She is not going back to Annecy!"

I managed to remind her that I had warned her of some possible alarming conduct on the part of her daughter, and pointed out that we had to meet to settle financial matters if the treatment were broken off, and that she could then tell me in person what had made her so angry. It took diplomacy, but I was able to arrange a meeting for that afternoon.

The mother arrived alone and still unhappy. I spoke first and calmly explained once again the possible problems of side effects, a problem which was a normal part of the treatment, but which she had brushed aside at our first discussion.

My visitor calmed down a little, and told me what had happened the day before.

"My parents, my in-laws and two couples who are friends of ours and their children came to dinner. We were at the table. The children were seated at the end of the table; they usually talk with each other without making too much noise, and talk to us only when asked to." In the middle of the meal, during a moment of silence, the daughter, in a loud voice and using the bluntest language, asked the mother a basic question about her father's anatomy. The guests and family could not believe that they had heard what they thought they had, and looked at each other in bewilderment. The girl repeated her question, with slightly different, but in no way improved, terminology. The father turned deep red and ordered her from the room.

The daughter answered with great calm, "I don't see, Papa, what's wrong with talking about things that are perfectly natural." She then got up and went to her room to sleep. The mother concluded by saying, "I leave to your imagination, Doctor, how the evening ended."

I repeated and amplified my explanations, but she was still somewhat dubious. She felt better once we had the daughter come in to go over the situation.

"Did you have a pleasant dinner yesterday?" I asked.

"Oh," the daughter answered simply, "I said a few dumb things and went to bed." The episode was clearly at an end, and the child had freed herself of a vocabulary accumulated through the years.

The last experience I shall touch on is that of an adult. The patient was a forty-five-year-old doctor who came to see me about some hearing problems. When I warned him about the possibility of a side effect, he answered with a big smile, "You know, my dear colleague, I am 80 kilos of good temper, mild as a lamb—it would take more than your pretty music to change that!"

I started the treatment, and every day my question would elicit the same answer: "No side effects?" "No, everything's fine."

One evening at the movies, I ran into the doctor and his

wife, who, after we were introduced, did not seem at all pleased to meet me. "Well, he's a nice bit of work, my husband, since you've been treating him!"

"Oh, you don't have to bring that up again," her husband said.

"Indeed I do! I'm telling you, you're unbearable these days, and there's no good reason for it."

I reminded the doctor that I had warned him of side effects and that he had reassured me that there were none.

His wife asked, "Has he told you that only the day before yesterday, after leaving you, he was so nervous that he demolished three cars leaving the parking lot? His own, the one that was blocking his way in front, and the one behind him!"

My colleague then admitted with a shamefaced laugh that he had not wanted to accept my warnings and explanations. His behavior problems ended on that day.

THE FOLLOW-UP EXAMINATION

At the beginning of this chapter, I mentioned the three-month follow-up; at least that amount of time is required before we could evaluate changes in behavior, at school or socially.

The reason is simple: normalization of behavior can be noticed at widely varying times, depending upon the patient. Conditions settle into normality over a length of time ranging from a few days to three months, rarely more, except with laterality problems. To avoid distressing parents, and the teachers who are waiting from day to day to see an improvement, we ask for an assessment only at the end of the third month.

If after this time, the results are not the ones that an improvement in hearing, as confirmed by the changes seen in the final audiogram, would lead us to expect, then another reason may be involved. It is often lack of effort on the part of the child, who may have decided that his improved hearing was enough to let him get good grades in school without extra work. This happens less and less often, because I am careful to explain to my young patients that good teeth are not enough to guarantee weight gain—one must also chew!

Chapter 7

CONCLUSION

THE HUMAN BEING is an extraordinarily complex entity.

The functioning of the human system calls for a harmonious interaction between its energy and each of its components. In a computer, the breakdown of a single element of the microprocessor can have catastrophic results. The same is true of the human body: the malfunctioning of one part, even a quite small one, can cause serious and unexpected problems.

It is a physician's duty to look for all possible causes of weakness, to find and identify them, and to remedy them wherever possible.

It seems apparent that malfunctioning of the auditory system, which so profoundly affects one's contact with the outside world, brings about such problems as dyslexia, depression and autism, among many others. The diagnosis and treatment of these auditory problems goes well beyond the traditional field of audiology, which has tended to see, and therefore find, comparatively simple sensory deficiencies.

During consultations or medical seminars, I am often faced with people saying, "Tell us about your method."

I disliked the possessive "your" in that request, because the vocation to treat, and sometimes to cure, is not something that can be owned. I came to accept its use, though, because I saw that my technique was unlike the one other therapists usually applied. I would say the difference arises from my refusal to eliminate from consideration facts and circumstances that seemed to contradict theory and previous information, or that failed to confirm what I thought to be the truth. That is how the pieces of the puzzle I found myself studying eventually fell into place.

Beyond "my" method, there exists a universal truth, which is that of the human body, of its physiology, of its failings, and of the simple observation of cause and effect in the relationship of an abnormality and an effect.

To arrive at this conclusion, one must know how to make decisions, and that is often extremely difficult. One must be receptive to information from all quarters, which means that one must be on guard against the often unconscious tendency to close the eyes, ears, and mind, believing that we have learned what there is to know on a topic. Barriers are so often erected by previous knowledge or by a ready-made way of doing things. The truth manages to emerge only when something new and unexpected can be fully exposed to study, discussion and argument, and accepted or refuted on that basis.

Once this principle is widely accepted, systematic research into auditory abnormalities throughout the full spectrum of frequencies will be possible. This research should be done widely enough so that a great number of audiograms and corresponding pathological records will be involved. Thanks to the "number crunching" capabilities of computers, we can now deal with very large amounts of information and explore this fascinating area more fully than was possible only a few years ago. I look forward to the development of more information on the medical problems I have discussed in this book, as well as on others whose origin is still unidentified.

It is not always possible to find the precise thing one is looking for, either in life in general or in science; but the search, conducted with a willingness to see what is there, is a never-ending adventure, with the richest of rewards.

PART TWO

Clinical Cases

CATEGORIES AND RESULTS

This section presents some of our experience with patients experiencing dyslexia, autism and depression or suicidal tendencies. Of the more than 8,000 auditory cases we have treated, about 2,300 fell into these categories, with results as follows:

• Dyslexia: 1,850 cases, 1,410 very positive results (76.2%), 440 noticeable partial improvement in one or more area (23.8%).

• Depression, suicidal tendencies: 233 cases, 217 cured after first course of treatment (93%), 11 healed after 2 or 3 treatments (4.7%), 4 failures after treatment, 1 suicide at beginning of treatment.

• Autism: 48 cases, 47 experienced disappearance of fear of noise, 47 had pronounced modification in behavior, 31 experienced progressive restoration or improvement of speech, 16 developed speech where it had not existed, 1 case experienced complete cure.

For each patient we show initial and post-treatment audiograms for each ear, allowing the reader with personal or professional interest in this field to see clearly the graphic images associated with the different sorts of problems, and those associated with the improved states described. The names given are of course false, to protect the patients' privacy, but are correct as to gender.

The symbols on the audiograms are:

← lateralization totally on the right for the frequency involved

→ lateralization totally on the left

○ no obvious lateralization on this frequency, or any frequencies

⊨ disturbed selection on all striped frequencies

// wrong selection only between the two frequencies shown

DYSLEXIA

Case No. 1

CHRISTOPHE

By the time he was thirteen, the difficulties in reading, writing and speech that had been with Christophe since preschool age had developed to such an extent that school work was impossible. Consultations with psychologists and pediatricians seemed to have had no useful effect, but a speech therapist had brought about some improvement.

The background information we obtained when he was brought to us in 1980 showed that his mother had had a difficult pregnancy with him and that he had severe otitis at the age of three (originating with a foreign object stuck in his nose that led to an infection of the eustachian tube).

The ENT examination showed no abnormalities. At the somatic examination we noticed that he had problems of balance and kicked with both feet, also that he wrote (poorly) with his left hand. It did not surprise us that the audiogram showed a totally disturbed lateralization, with quick answers on the left and slow answers on the right, with retention; there were also hyperaudition peaks at 4,000 Hz in both ears.

The treatment produced reactions of fatigue during the first days and periods of nervousness toward the end. As can be seen from the lower charts, the hearing abnormalities were removed, resulting in a line very close to the flat line of absolute perfection, including almost perfect lateralization.

We considered this audiogram to be predictive of good results, and so it was. The three-month report showed excellent progress from the beginning, and special achievements in English, in which he had been doing quite poorly.

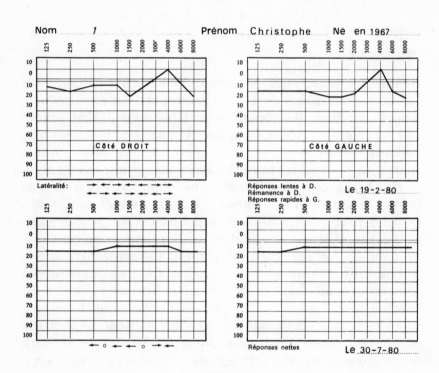

FIGURE D-1

Case No. 2

AMÉLIE

Amélie was brought to us at the age of eight, in October 1971 on the advice of the last of a series of doctors and psychologists her family had consulted. Her speech was so poor that even her brothers could not understand what she was trying to say.

There was nothing in Amélie's family history to supply a clue to her problem. She had experienced some childhood problems, such as a bout of false croup before her first birthday, followed by a period of separation from her family, with subsequent evidence of depression, and, at three, a fall from a balcony, resulting in her isolation for a month. The most significant experience from our point of view was recurrent earache for several years; these ceased when her adenoids were removed when she was five.

Amélie's consultation disclosed in her left ear a buildup of wax, which we removed, and crossed body lateralization—sound frequencies received differently in each ear. The audiogram showed a hearing loss of 25 percent in her right ear and distortions on the left, and that the right ear was receiving lower frequency sounds and the left ear the higher frequencies.

The treatment to address these conditions was not difficult to prepare, and was administered uneventfully, though Amélie appeared somewhat nervous around the tenth session. The post-treatment audiogram showed that all hearing abnormalities had disappeared, and that the lateralization had gone completely to the right.

We did not see for ourselves the long-term results of the treatment, but letters from Amélie's parents indicated that it had been highly successful. Four months after she had completed the treatment, her mother wrote that all was well and that "a new life starts for my daughter."

After two years, the mother wrote that "this child is now blossoming at all levels, and this is quite spectacular in relation to the state she was in when we brought her to you. . . . Her personality has developed quite a lot. She expresses

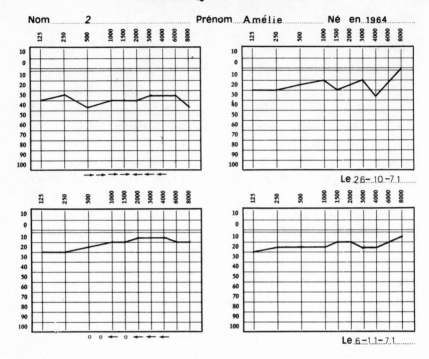

FIGURE D-2

herself better.... She reads with greater pleasure ... withstands fatigue better. Her movements have more coordination."

A final letter, ten years after the treatment, let us know that the news about Amélie was still excellent.

Case No. 3

ALICE

Alice was immensely shy when she came to us at the age of twelve, referred by a psychologist friend of her family; she utterly lacked self-confidence and was having a difficult time in school, finding it particularly hard to move on from one subject to another; her spelling was extremely poor.

The only item of possible relevance in her history was that the umbilical cord had been wrapped around her at birth, but that seemed to have created no discernible problem.

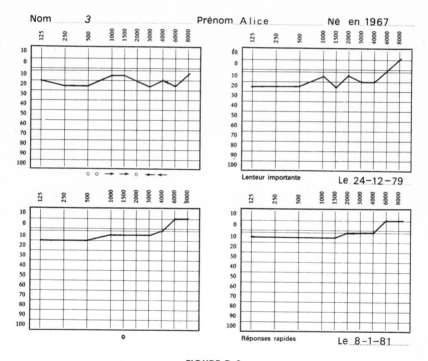

FIGURE D-3

Her ENT and physical examinations showed normal conditions. Audiograms showed bilateral distortions and crossed lateralization. The slowness of her answers had a pretty obvious connection to her school problems. The left-ear peaks at 1,000, 2,000 and 8,000 Hz often manifest, in children of this age, as shyness and avoidance of social contact.

During the treatment Alice was tired for the first three days, then roused herself to play tricks on her family, and, toward the end, showed considerable excitement. The treatment eliminated the abnormalities, and after-treatment evaluation disclosed noticeable progress in reading, math and homework, and the referring psychologist observed an improvement in behavior. Her spelling stayed quite as bad as it had been, though.

Case No. 4

ANTONIO

Antonio started life traumatically, with encephalopathy and consequent blood transfusion at birth; then, three months later, he developed a pulmonary infection that required two hospital stays.

At fifteen, a student in a Montessori school, his I.Q. tested at 40. He was referred to me by his doctor in Italy.

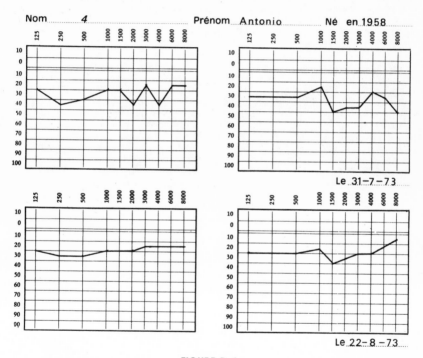

Nom _4_ Prénom _Antonio_ Né en 1958

Le 31-7-73

Le 22-8-73

FIGURE D-4

The audiogram showed important distortions and substantial hypohearing; i.e., hearing nothing at the 10 dB level and only starting to hear around 20 or 30 dB.

He showed no reactions to the treatment at first, but developed some nervousness and impatience after the tenth session. The final audiogram showed a flattening of the line, and a diminishing, though not removal, of the hearing loss. This led us to expect a general improvement, and the parents indeed reported it, noting that Antonio had become "happy and affectionate."

Case No. 5

NICOLAS

This eight-year-old had not begun to speak until the age of two and a half, and had problems in school, mainly of confusion among the letters. There was no way of knowing if his need of an oxygen mask at birth had any connection with his condition.

Nicolas's ENT examination was normal; his audiogram displayed dyslaterality, and a perfectly functioning right ear matched with 1-2-8 distortions on the left.

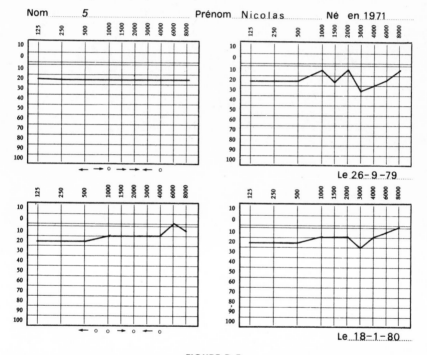

FIGURE D-5

This seemed a case that might be treated with medication, but another audiogram eight weeks later showed no change, and we elected to start auditory retraining. Nicolas was very excited and aggressive during both the day and the night at the beginning of the treatment, but quieted down after the tenth session. His mother reported that he seemed to understand better.

The final audiogram showed disappearance of distortions and almost total lateralization on the right. Positive results could be expected from this, and the family's detailed report three months later described a complete cure.

Case No. 6

CHRISTIAN

At six, Christian did not seem to like anyone, neither such friends as he had nor his parents. There was the possibility of a birth trauma, and the certainty that he had been quite late starting to speak and to walk.

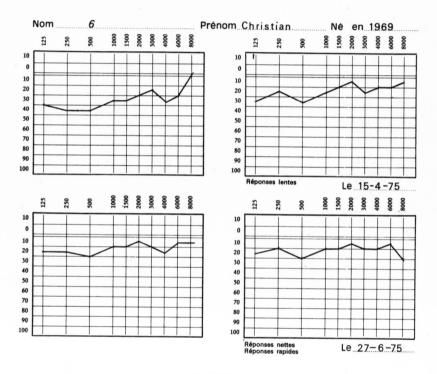

FIGURE D-6

The audiogram showed a severe loss of hearing on the right, strong bilateral distortion, and a slight 2-8 curve on the left, well short of the indicators of dangerous depression.

During treatment, Christian carried on wildly for the first week, then became quieter. The post-treatment audiogram showed a leveling of the lines; another encouraging sign was that his answers were clear and quick.

The prognosis was good, and later reports showed him as doing excellently in school and in behavior, and, as his parents put it, "happy and blossoming."

Case No. 7

CATHERINE

According to her parents, nervous teachers and troubled relationships with her two sisters were at the root of Catherine's problems in school, including aggressiveness toward other children; but one might better consider the probable childhood otitis and the adenoid removal at the age of eight. Whatever the cause, she was also late in developing speech.

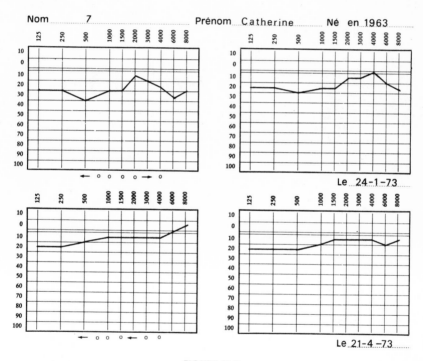

FIGURE D-7

The audiogram showed bilateral distortion, especially on the right, and dips at 500 Hz in both ears (bilateral scotome), which is associated with aggressiveness.

This trait did not show up during treatment; instead Catherine experienced deep fatigue at the outset, which lifted somewhat later on. The treatment resulted in a virtually perfect audiogram, prompting hope for improvement in school as well as in relationships.

The results were in fact highly positive, and defined as a success by the family. Catherine's aggressiveness disappeared and her psychological equilibrium was excellent. She had been poor at foreign language study; now she did well, and developed a taste for reading; and in fact moved from the lowest scholastic grouping in her class to the highest.

Case No. 8

BERTRAND

Bertrand seemed to have no problems during the first four years of his life. Then teachers and parents noticed a worrisome constant sadness; Bertrand did not smile or play any more. His father, a psychologist, could establish neither a reason for the situation nor a solution to it.

When we saw him, we were shocked by the fixed expression of sadness and fatigue on this five-year-old's face, a marked contrast to his older sister. The audiogram showed a few bilateral distortions and a troubling, exceptional 1-2-8 curve on the right.

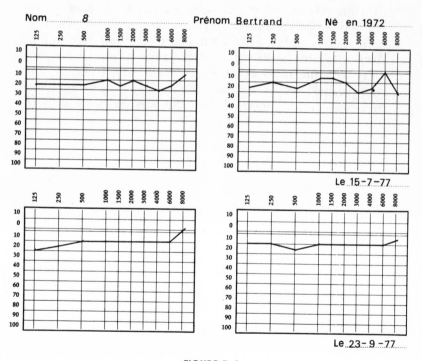

FIGURE D-8

Bertrand displayed many reactions during the retraining, starting with deep fatigue after the first six sessions. Then, after eight sessions, things moved quickly: Bertrand began to smile; the next day he laughed; the day after, he was singing with his sister. After the fourteenth session, we had a friendly demon who laughed and played jokes on his adult neighbors in the retraining room; he would make the most horrible faces at us, then wave and blow kisses. In short, a magnificent and sudden improvement!

The final audiogram was nearly perfect, and, with the changes Bertrand had shown during treatment, suggested an excellent prognosis.

A letter from the father confirmed this:

> My unhappy, introverted, mocked and defenseless son . . . all that disappeared after our stay in Annecy.
>
> Smiles, even laughter, ease in his movements as well as with his relationships. His behavior has no lack of humor, and we, as well as our friends, are constantly surprised.
>
> In short, the boy is blooming. School interests him a lot. And as for his bouts with anxiety, they seem to have flown away with the musical tones you made him listen to. Even when he asks us about death, the explanations we give seem to relieve him, whereas before he was obsessed with this topic.

Case No. 9

ARNAUD

Arnaud was a little bit later than the norm in teething, walking and speaking, and experienced episodes of severe otitis between the ages of two and five, once requiring surgical drainage of fluid (paracentesis) from the affected area. He experienced a wide range of classroom and social problems from the beginning of his school days, and was finally referred to us by a physician at the age of fourteen.

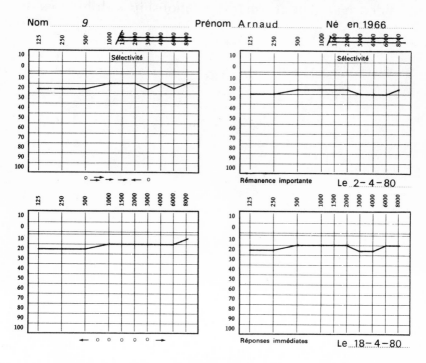

FIGURE D-9

The ENT examination showed a significant deviation in the nasal cavity. The audiogram showed a slight loss of hearing with high-frequency sounds, poor bilateral selection, and dominant left lateralization. Retention (inability to note precisely the instant of the ending of sound transmission) was particularly marked. Arnaud was extremely sleepy after the treatment sessions.

The final audiogram was excellent, though a slight lateralization problem persisted; selectivity was normalized, and the retention completely disappeared. All this boded well for improvement in school.

At the end of the school year, Arnaud's performance in all his subjects had improved, and his scholastic average had risen from 7.7 points (out of a possible 20) to 13. All behavior problems disappeared, and he has developed self-confidence and an affirmative relationship with his friends.

Case No. 10

GILLES

Like Arnaud, Gilles had had otitis requiring paracentesis, an episode involving both ears when he was three, as well as removal of his adenoids at four, and was subject to inflammations of the nose and pharynx. His difficulties in school, including his tendency to spell phonetically (e.g., "funettiklee"), led to his dropping out of school for technical training. He came to us at the age of seventeen from a specialized center where he was being taken care of.

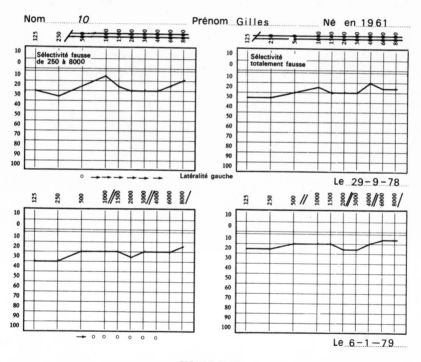

FIGURE D-10

The first audiogram showed strong distortions, with no selectivity—practically all frequencies were affected—and total lateralization on the left.

After treatment, during which Gilles showed no notable reactions, the distortions disappeared, selectivity was improved, and the left lateralization disappeared, leading to a favorable prognosis.

After four months, the special center reported good results, with no more phonetic spelling, and many sentences being written without a mistake.

Case No. 11

HERVÉ

Hervé was brought to us at the age of eleven by the director of the private school he attended because he felt that this child, brilliant in every area, was not using his skills to the maximum, and that he panicked easily and became discouraged quickly.

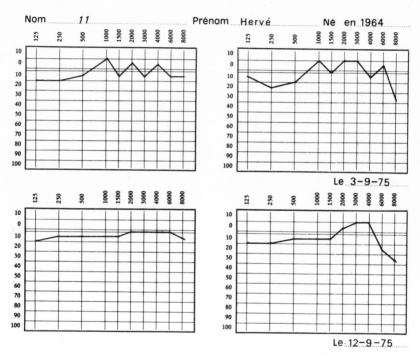

FIGURE D-11

The audiogram for the right ear showed a saw-toothed line indicating considerable distortion; there was some loss of hearing at 8,000 Hz in the right ear. We first tried medical treatment, but after four months we saw no change, and recommended retraining.

Throughout its course, Hervé seemed irritable, and complained of stomachache. The final audiogram showed a perfect right ear and a slight persistence of the high-frequency hearing loss on the left.

The favorable prognosis this suggested was borne out by a letter from the parents reporting that the boy was doing well.

Case No. 12

CHARLOTTE

Charlotte's tonsils and adenoids were removed when she was ten, three years before she was brought to us because of her problems in adapting to school, and particularly in spelling; she also had recurring spells of sadness. Treatment for her dyslexia had not been effective, as our initial examination verified.

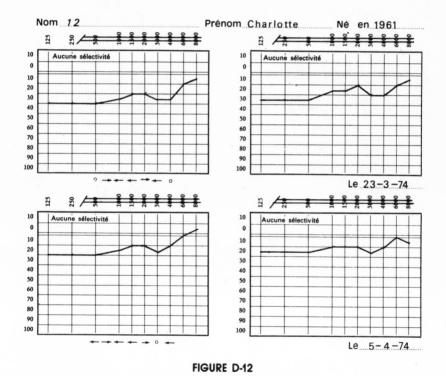

FIGURE D-12

The audiogram showed poor transmission at 2,000 and 8,000 Hz on the left, general dyslexia and no selectivity. During the treatment, Charlotte slept most of the day.

Treatment resulted in the removal of the distortions and the 2-8 curve, but there were no changes in the selectivity and dyslexia. The prognosis was for behavioral improvement, with the disappearance of the 2-8 curve, but not for any improvement in school work. Her parents later reported that Charlotte was a good bit happier, and had opened up to friendship and social relationships, but was doing no better in school.

Case No. 13

SIMONE

Simone was a slow student, getting average marks only by making a tremendous effort. At the age of nine, she was seeing a psychiatrist for bouts of depression. She was born after a difficult pregnancy threatened by miscarriage, and had a few episodes of otitis followed by chronic pharyngitis.

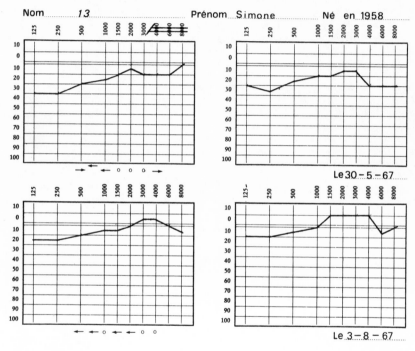

FIGURE D-13

The initial audiogram showed that both of Simone's ears heard low frequencies poorly, resulting in poor perception of voiceless consonants. She also had a slight 2-8 curve on the right, and crossed lateralization.

During the treatment she showed no unpleasant reactions, but in fact was calmer, more content and more inclined to work, and was no longer depressed. The audiogram showed great improvement, with the disappearance of the 2-8 curve and lateralization switched to the right side.

A few weeks later, Simone's mother told me she had improved in all areas—hearing, work, personality and vocabulary. A checkup a year and a half later showed perfect hearing and excellent work at school.

Case No. 14

FRANCIS

A doctor's son, Francis put even more effort than Simone
into school work, and achieved less, obtaining only barely
acceptable results. His parents brought him to us for evaluation when he was fourteen.

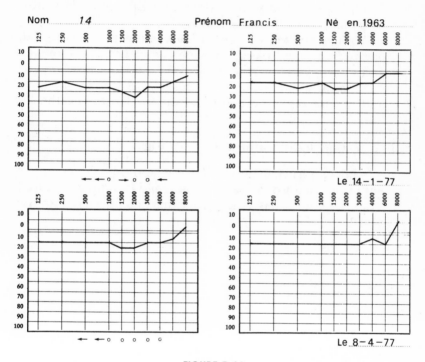

FIGURE D-14

The somatic examination showed a bodily dyslaterality.
The audiogram revealed moderately important distortions,
especially in the region of the "whistling" sounds, and a
slight dyslaterality.

The audiogram taken after treatment showed the distortions to be almost completely gone, and complete lateralization to the right, adding up to a highly positive prognosis.

I had two letters from the parents, the first two months
after the completion of treatment:

Our child is going to finish the school year this coming week, but we can tell you the results now.

Dictation is his weakest area, but he has brought his work up to an average level. His French teacher has commented on a language improvement.

In German, he will receive a passing grade for the first time since he began to study it, three years ago.

Even though it is less than three months since the treatment, improvements are obvious enough to allow Francis to be promoted to the next grade.

We look for even more striking results this coming fall, because our child has gained self-confidence and shows eagerness in everything he does.

As far as we are concerned, this is what matters the most, and we are deeply grateful to you for having set the kid "straight."

The second letter came the following year:

School improvements are so great, and this with no apparent effort, that we can say that our child is completely cured. Your treatment has reached its full potential after only a year.

One conclusion to be drawn from this case is that even a slight auditory abnormality can be enough to block a child's intellectual potential.

Case No. 15

JEAN-PIERRE

Jean-Pierre's dyslexia was diagnosed as soon as he entered school, and treated since then, without much result up to the age of twelve; he had also had speech therapy.

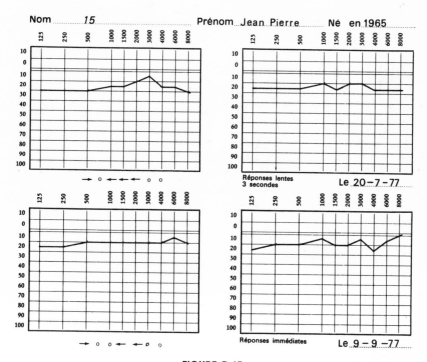

FIGURE D-15

The ENT examination showed a severe allergic rhinitis. The audiogram showed a light distortion on the right, with the frequency at 3,000 Hz tending to mask the others. Jean-Pierre's response time was extremely slow, about three seconds instead of one or less.

The reaction the treatment elicited was aggressive behavior toward his sister. The results, as shown in the last

audiogram, were normalization of the right ear and restoration of normal response time.

Evaluation after treatment confirmed the expected disappearance of his dyslexia.

AUTISM

Case No. 1

KAREN

Karen came to us from America, preceded by an extensive file sent by the League for the Hard of Hearing in New York. From this I excerpt some relevant information:

- At the age of eight months, she suffered a severe viral otitis, after which her parents noticed a change in behavior, particularly a developmental regression.
- At 21 months, she had a vocabulary of ten words; after neurological and psychiatric examinations, she was labeled as autistic, and placed in a specialized school.
- At the age of 31 months, it became evident that she feared some loud sounds.
- When she was three, she had a tonsillectomy and tracheotomy.

The adorable, affectionate, smiling child I saw in my office was ten years old, but spoke on the level of a three- or four-year-old, and at times seemed "out of it." I had to clap my hands or touch her in order to get her attention.

Autistic children can be difficult to examine, but Karen presented no problems with the ENT (which showed a slight rhinitis) or the audiogram, which showed very pronounced bilateral distortions.

We did not test to see if strong intensities caused pain, fearing to risk a negative reaction against the earphones and the treatment itself.

Treatment was started with no problems, and Karen came to the sessions willingly, but would rapidly become

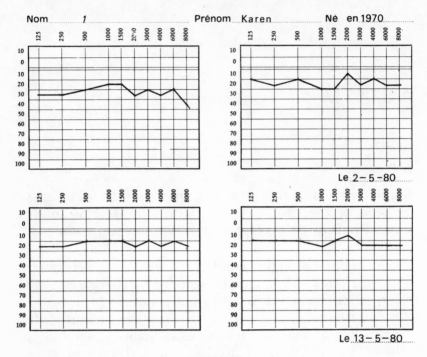

FIGURE A-1

aggressive toward her mother, hitting her hard while smiling broadly. The final audiogram was almost perfect—and, unusually, the normalization was achieved half-way through the treatment, and observed on the midpoint audiogram taken then.

The parents sent me a three-page report some months after treatment; here are some comments from it:

> Many changes have taken place since last year. The first thing we noticed is that she is no longer afraid of violent noises. . . .
>
> We saw right away that she could understand a lot better. Her answers to our questions are quicker and more understandable. I can't say that she understands everything, because sometimes her answers are still confused.
>
> . . . She seems more alert, and, on her own, she seems to want to participate in activities around her. This happened

soon after your treatment, and she had certainly not been like that before.

. . . Her inversions of numbers and letters have decreased but not disappeared.

I might note here that, for reasons I have already mentioned, a good proportion of my autistic patients have come from the United States; and it happens that all the cases I shall describe here are of American children.

Case No. 2

PATRICIA

Patricia seems to have had problems since birth, as shown in the complete and detailed report sent to us by her mother and by two specialized institutions. She presented an unusual case, difficult to diagnose specifically, such as apraxia, ataxia or autism. The earliest problems noticed were in feeding and stability; then some motor retardation was seen when she was ready to walk, followed by slow psychomotor development. Later it was noticed that she did not learn to speak, and had frequent destructive temper tantrums. By the age of ten, it seemed that she understood what was said to her, but expressed herself only through gestures and a few garbled words.

Patricia was pretty, with an expressive face, and made no bother over the ENT examination, but it was impossible to obtain an audiogram; as I explained in the chapter on autism, you cannot get an audiogram with a nonverbal subject, so we were compelled to limit our treatment to dealing with the ascertainable problem of frequencies and intensities that produced discomfort, and gearing the auditory training to them.

During this process, Patricia was very aggressive, particularly toward her mother, and, in the early days, suffered from insomnia. And, of course, no final audiogram was possible.

Obviously, without the ability to diagnose or treat Patricia fully, it was difficult to estimate what the result of the partial treatment we had been able to give would be.

After five months, some positive results were evident. Patricia had improved as follows:

- showed greater interest in people around her
- increased attention span
- better participation in group activities
- noticeable improvement and integration into everyday life

- expressed feelings of affection
- strong reduction in destructive tendencies.

On the negative side, she had no improvement in the area of speech. These results were confirmed after two years.

Case No. 3

EDWARD

Edward, eleven years old, did not present a case of true autism, but a serious behavioral abnormality. He had many episodes of otitis in rapid succession: at 6 months, 9 months, 14 months and so on, but was otherwise in good health.

He had acquired speech only with great labor, a few words by two, some sentence fragments at three, and now, at ten, spoke little and with difficulty. From the age of two he had been afraid of loud noises, enough so that he would scream, run away or hide under a table.

When Edward was five and a half, he was labeled retarded and put in a specialized school, where the staff took note of his neurological immaturity and poor coordination. The teachers insisted that he had auditory dysfunction, and also that he was hyperactive and anxious, with a tendency to fantasize.

At the initial examination, the boy projected stubbornness and hostility. He pulled his head into his shoulders, and looked at us sidelong if at all. I was able, though, to take an audiogram, and this showed important distortions, a drop in hearing acuity at 500 Hz in both ears, and dyslateralization.

For the first four days of training, Edward showed some anger, occasionally violent, and seemed to express fear over the next retraining session. After that, things smoothed out, and we were suddenly dealing with a pleasant, smiling boy who had his picture taken with my secretary and did what everyone assured me was an amazingly accurate imitation of me.

The final audiogram was excellent, almost perfect, and I felt happy about making a positive prognosis. A letter nine months later gave the picture, mainly positive but with a few negative elements. Some excerpts:

> Edward's behavior shows great improvement socially, emotionally and at school. He has much more self-confidence. Before the treatment, he always walked with his head down.

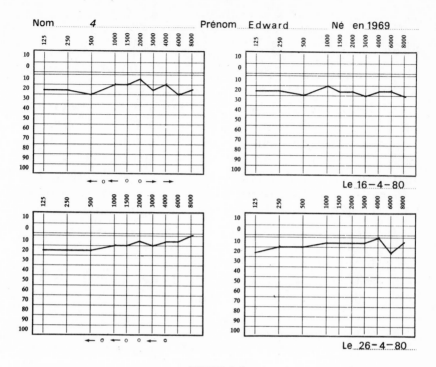

FIGURE A-2

But by the middle of the treatment, he was walking upright, and still is. . . .

He is no longer passive and asserts himself a lot better. This has posed a problem, because now he argues with his brother, but this seems on the whole positive to us. On his first day of school in September, a friend of his who used to pick on him without getting any reaction, was surprised when he tried it and was thrown by a Judo move. There have been no provocateurs since that day.

He understands and answers rapidly. . . . He expresses himself better. . . . He is much more relaxed at school. . . . much improved memory . . . progress in reading . . .

On the other hand, there is no improvement as far as his fantasies are concerned. He has frightening visions, and this gives him feelings of guilt. This problem should be looked into.

HUGH

Hugh manifested no problems until the age of 21 months, when he still could not walk. Testing at the age of three showed negative results in a variety of mental and developmental areas, and he was placed in a specialized school for retarded children, then in a school for autism. An audiometric examination showed no hearing loss, but was impeded by the child's screams and his severe agitation. The report sent by his parents showed that some sounds made him cry and cover his ears with his hands. He was not steadily angry, but yelled when he was refused something. His vocabulary consisted of only a few words, reserved for when he had some demand to make.

In spite of this history, Hugh showed himself to be a quiet child, affectionate, and easy to do the ENT examination on—and, as might be expected, impossible when it came to the audiogram.

The limited treatment we were able to do produced strong results during its course. His parents reported an improvement "at all levels," and claimed at the end of the ten days that he now had an excellent sense of direction and showed some understanding of cause and effect as it related to behavior.

The parents some months later sent us a long, detailed letter containing only good news:

> The reason for this long delay in giving you any information is that there was so much progress that we are always waiting for more before writing to you. Hugh's speech has become much clearer, and he is using organized sentences. . . .
>
> This summer he has started to ride a bike and play ball, and goes to the pool, where he is learning to swim. Watches television and can stay in front of it without moving from his seat during the whole length of the program. . . .
>
> At school, he is learning to read, spell and count. His speech therapist notices a great improvement. . . .
>
> In conclusion, all of his teachers feel that Hugh is doing remarkably well. As far as I am concerned, there is so much improvement that I am thrilled beyond words.

Case No. 5

HUBERT

Hubert's family background included a deaf grandfather and a dyslexic older brother. At the age of three, he had made a few chattering sounds but not reached the stage of imitating sounds; at this time he was diagnosed as autistic at New York University Medical Center's Department of Psychiatry. After that he was sent to special schools.

When he was six, an examination at the New York League for the Hard of Hearing confirmed the earlier diagnosis. The audiometric examination was impossible, but it was noticed that whenever a sound "too loud is sent out, the child would start to scream, the examination would go on for a moment, and then he would cry out again, even at sounds of lesser intensity. . . . A great amount of time during the examination was spent on the floor with the child screaming and covering his ears with his hands."

The testing doctor's conclusion was that there was no hearing loss or over-hearing. I concur, and believe that the observed actions were the result of painful hearing.

In Annecy as well as New York, the audiogram could not be obtained, and we set about treating the painful hearing. Hubert showed some agitation during sleep, but after the twentieth session, his mother reported that his walk was more confident, he smiled more and seemed more coordinated, and he made a variety of noises and used a few words. We decided that this was one of the rare cases in which extending treatment past the standard twenty sessions would be productive, and went on for a dozen more.

The results were not spectacular. Hubert was calmer and less noisy. He understood his environment better, and used short words more frequently, but still had difficulty with consonants.

After about a year, the improvement appeared to stop, and we decided on another course of treatment. Reactions observed during this were nervousness, increased appetite, and a tendency to use new phonemes. The results of this treatment were insignificant.

Case No. 7

NELLY

For this seven-year-old we received a report of about 60 pages, which included medical as well as school information. Some salient points:

- For the hereditary component, there were auditory problems in the father's family.
- Nelly showed no problems in early infancy, with normal development of speech at 12 months; about this time she experienced numerous infections of the inner ear.
- At 14 months, her language capacity disappeared, and she showed fits of jealousy at the birth of a sister.
- She developed slowly for a year, and since her speech did not return, she was examined at Harvard Medical School and diagnosed as autistic, at the age of three.
- In the special school she was sent to, she manifested anguish, a tendency to solitude, general motor awkwardness and jerky movements, and very slow progress in speech.
- Her father commented several times on her fear of loud sounds. "She has always reacted with fear to sudden loud noises (popping balloons, thunder, etc.) with fearful movements and by covering her ears."

This last went with the fact that painful hearing was the only problem we could treat, in the absence of any possibility of taking an audiogram. During the treatment Nelly showed early aggressiveness and was quite bossy with her family. In a short while we could see an improvement in speech, and she came happily to the retraining sessions. Toward the middle of the treatment, she reported some episodes of stomach pain. At the end of treatment, she showed a persistent nervousness, and seemed not to like the idea of returning to the U.S.

The report we had a year later indicated excellent general results.

REMARKS ON AUTISTIC CHILDREN

The failure noted at the end of Hubert's second treatment, which was also observed in two other identical cases, prompts me to make the following observations:

1) The contribution of an auditory problem to autism seems absolutely certain, because all the children we treated for such problems experienced some improvement. These improvements were in behavior or speech, or both.

2) The auditory problem, however, cannot be considered the only cause of autism, because, even when the ear has been normalized, some symptoms are still present, to an extent that varies with each individual.

It would seem, then, that hearing is only a part of the problem, as far as autism is concerned; but this is not absolutely certain. In my opinion, the matter can be looked at in this simplified way:

• either, at the onset of the condition, there was a hearing deficiency plus something else; or
• the origin of the problem is purely auditory, and the malfunctions it produces in the brain remain through the years, becoming irreversible even if the auditory problems are later normalized.

Which of these alternative hypotheses is true can perhaps be best determined by systematic treatment of autism with auditory training as soon as the illness is diagnosed. The ultimate effectiveness of this treatment in a large number of cases, would provide evidence to answer the question. The likelihood that the second hypothesis is correct seems strong in those cases in which the parents report that autism developed after the child suffered infections of the middle ear.

DEPRESSION, WITH SUICIDAL TENDENCIES

Case No. 1

BRIGITTE

Brigitte, child of an extremely difficult birth, had been obsessed with death since the age of five, and, eleven years later, when her mother brought her to us, would answer any question the same way: "I want to die."

She had expected not to live past twelve; when she survived, she had a romance, which broke up and led to a persistent depression and visits to various specialized establishments, where the strongest medication produced no positive results.

Her desperate parents consulted a doctor in Geneva, who referred them to me. Her mother, in tears, said that Brigitte's wish for death was her only topic of conversation between hospital stays, and that she had twice actually attempted suicide.

I had seen enough such patients to expect what I found on the initial audiogram, the sensitivity at 2,000 and 8,000 Hz—the 2-8 curve—in the left ear.

During retraining, Brigitte showed extreme fatigue, especially after the morning sessions, and each "How are you today?" brought the answer, "I want to die." The checkup audiogram after the tenth session showed some improvement, but her attitude did not.

After the fourteenth session, Brigitte underwent a sudden metamorphosis: the sad creature, careless of dress, became a young lady with a nice hairdo, wearing a charming flowered-print dress. Her mother still cried, but with joy.

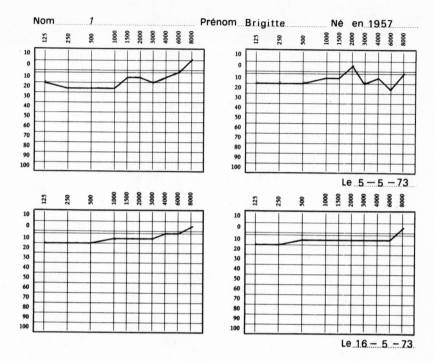

FIGURE Dp-1

The final audiogram was perfect, and prompted us to feel highly hopeful. As soon as Brigitte was back home, she sought ways to work to become useful, and physical and mental anticipation replaced her depression. An audiogram two and a half years later confirmed that the hearing normalization persisted.

Case No. 2

GUY

There were hearing problems on his mother's side of the family, but Guy did not manifest any such condition. In school, his grades seesawed between satisfactory and deplorable, and in the 11th grade he dropped his studies and entered art school. For a year, he felt despondent and harbored suicidal thoughts, but made no actual attempts. He saw a psychologist, with whom, as he put it, "nothing was happening." At nineteen, he was brought to us for consultation.

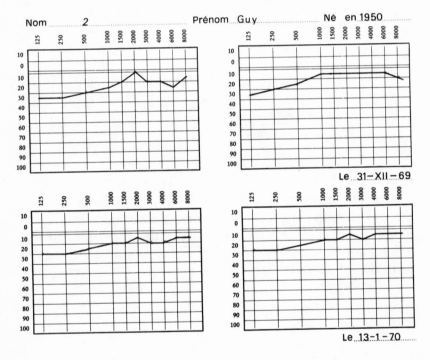

FIGURE Dp-2

His ENT examination showed a malformation of the nasal septum which called for an operation. The audiogram showed the standard suicidal 2-8 curve, but on the right.

Guy experienced only one strong reaction during treatment, a feeling of being filled with an intense joy after the third session. The final audiogram showed disappearance of the 2-8 curve, leading us to hope for full recovery. After-treatment evaluation confirmed this, and a letter ten years later showed that the cure appeared to be permanent.

Case No. 3

ETIENNE

Etienne was sent to us at the age of twenty-nine by a colleague who was worried about his chronic depression and tendency to cut off and withdraw from social contact, and who knew that standard treatments—and even some non-standard ones—had not helped.

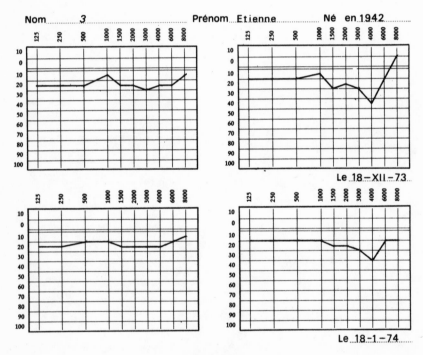

FIGURE Dp-3

The consultation confirmed this. From the beginning of treatment, Etienne reported feeling happier, and also told us of strange feelings in his ears and that they didn't seem to be working harmoniously. After the fourteenth session, this feeling seemed to disappear completely, and he told us he felt fine.

The final audiogram showed considerable improvement, and we felt confident that the suicidal tendency would disappear. It did so, and a letter a year later confirmed that it had not returned.

Case No. 4

BÉATRICE

At the age of thirty-six, Béatrice was assailed by a feeling of depression coupled with a wish to kill herself. She resisted this sufficiently to seek treatment for it, but without result.

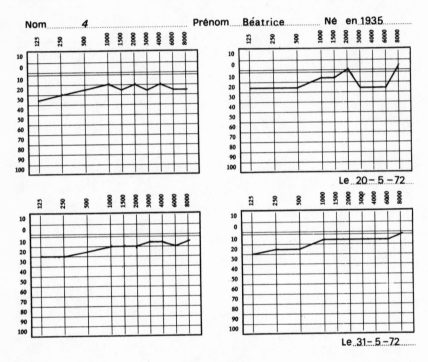

FIGURE Dp-4

The audiogram showed the predictable 2-8 curve on the left. As soon as we began treatment, Béatrice told us that she felt better. The ninth and tenth sessions seemed to exhaust her totally, but this lasted only a day, and then steady improvement continued to the end of treatment.

The final audiogram was just about perfect. Four months later, Béatrice was living a normal life. She experienced brief regressions two and three years later, and each time the audiogram showed the 2-8 curve on the left, proving that the improvements we had obtained with the twenty treatments were only transitory.

We tried two more series of treatments, twenty sessions each, and hoped they would do the job. They appeared to, as we have kept in touch with Béatrice and her suicidal tendency seems to have disappeared for good, and the 2-8 curve has not recurred.

Case No. 5

EDITH

At twenty-nine, Edith was in a state of near-permanent depression, and had a history of serious suicide attempts. Her father was partially deaf, and she had several episodes of otitis in infancy, and had "never felt quite right." The year before she came to us, she was hospitalized in a clinic for sleep treatment, without much effect.

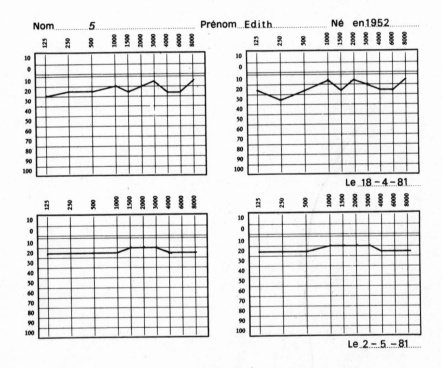

FIGURE Dp-5

The ENT examination showed large pieces of ear wax, which we removed immediately. The audiogram showed the 1-2-8 curve on the left, the clear indicator of suicidal depression, and a few distortions on the right.

During treatment, Edith showed two nervous reactions, and experienced first insomnia and then drowsiness.

Her final audiogram was perfect, leading to a very favorable prognosis. Later evaluation suggested a total cure.

Case No. 6

ELISABETH

Lucky Elisabeth! She insisted that she had no problems at home, she got on well with her husband and three children, there were no financial worries, and at thirty-eight, she had every reason to be happy.

All the same, she had numerous spells of depression, none the less severe for not having a "sensible" cause, the usual treatments did no good, and she eventually came to consult us.

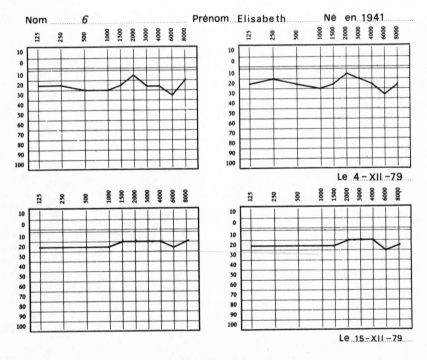

FIGURE Dp-6

Elisabeth's audiogram showed a bilateral 2-8 curve. She was nervous and aggressive during the early stages of treatment, and also slept better, though insomnia set in after the last sessions. Her post-treatment audiogram was almost perfect, and the favorable prognosis turned out to be amply justified when she remained well and happy.

Case No. 7

NORBERT

Norbert did well in school; but at the age of twenty-one, following a severe problem at home, he developed a nervous depression which pretty much immobilized him. Psychoanalysis and narcoleptic treatment were not effective. Following a serious crisis, he was hospitalized in a special ward and eventually referred to us by a physician.

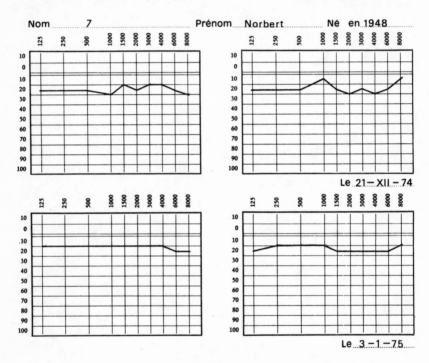

FIGURE Dp-7

The important 1-8 curve on the left displayed by the audiogram fit the clinical picture smoothly. Beginning with the first sessions, Norbert told us of a feeling of relaxation that increased as the treatment progressed. The final audiogram was very good, and the prognosis favorable.

Post-treatment evaluation showed improvement lasting six months, followed by a regression and confinement in a psychiatric hospital. A new examination after a year showed an audiogram identical to the pre-treatment one. Again, a twenty-session retraining program was undertaken, occasioning reactions that went up and down: improvement for two days, then regression, then improvement again.

The final audiogram was perfect, and a checkup six months later showed that Norbert seemed to have recovered.

Case No. 8

ODILE

Odile had frequent otitis during infancy, but now, more than thirty years later, the constant violent headaches and pervasive depression were far heavier problems. The impressive variety of drugs prescribed for the depression did not seem to be doing much good, even though she was swallowing ten kinds of pills each day.

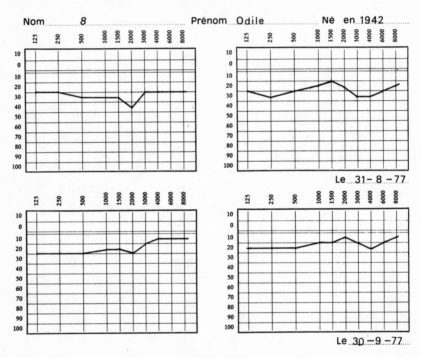

FIGURE Dp-8

The audiogram showed a 1.5-8 curve on the left and a slight impairment on the right. At the beginning of treatment she showed brief spells of aggressiveness, and then was in a generally nervous state until the treatment was over. The headaches that had hit her every day for two weeks before she came to Annecy vanished, and she almost completely suspended her medication.

154

The final audiogram was almost perfect except for the minimal 2-8 curve remaining on the left, leading to a cautious prognosis.

After three months there was solid improvement, but Odile still suffered from insomnia. Seven months later she experienced a sudden regression after a stay in the mountains, and a new audiogram was worse than the first. We were about to suggest urgently a new series of treatments, but Odile requested it first.

The reactions were stronger than the first time, aggressiveness followed by headaches. The audiogram was again good, and the patient seemed settled.

There was another regression after two years, and the 2-8 curve reappeared on the audiogram, this time in both ears.

The third course of treatment was accompanied by painful stomachaches after almost all sessions. The third audiogram was perfect, and Odile's depressive state disappeared and has not recurred.

Case No. 9

ISABELLE

The case of this charming young woman, whose problems went back six years, interested us tremendously, because the audiometric evolution was undulating and symptomatic.

There was nothing especially remarkable or troubling in Isabelle's life until, at the age of twenty-eight, a deep state of depression overcame her. It was treated with the usual variety of drugs, and her condition improved. Then, after six years, she suffered a new depression without any apparent reason, as she claimed to feel perfectly content in all aspects of her life.

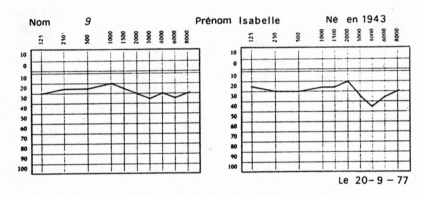

FIGURE Dp-9

Isabelle came to see us on the recommendation of a friend who had once been our patient. The audiogram (Figure Dp-9) showed a 2-8 on the left, aggravated by a slight 1-8 on the right.

During the eighth session of treatment, some irritability appeared, then pain in the ears, then insomnia. The audiometric curve was modified after the tenth session (Figure Dp-10).

The 2-8 on the left had become a 1-8, and the 1-8 on the right had changed its appearance. During the second part of the treatment, Odile experienced a liver attack

156

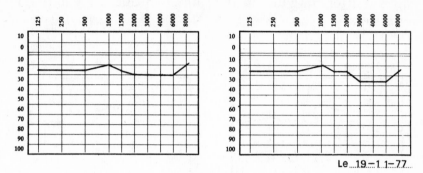

FIGURE Dp-10.

which lasted a few days. She stopped taking medication, her own idea, and slept better.

The post-treatment audiogram (Figure Dp-11) showed the absence of any depressive abnormality on the left, but the 1-8 on the right was worse. We decided, unless something unexpected happened, to do a checkup at the end of four months. The unexpected did happen two months later, a slight state of depression toward six every day, accompanied by some digestive problems.

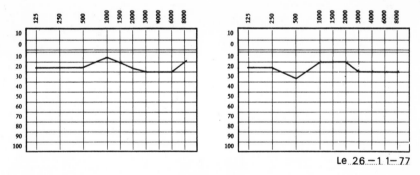

FIGURE Dp-11

The checkup done at that point confirmed the setback, with a 1-2-8 on the left and a persistent 1-8 on the right (Figure Dp-12).

The treatment started more than a month later and, very

rapidly after fatigue at the outset, Isabelle's condition improved.

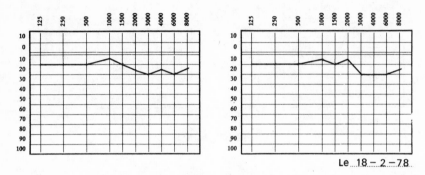

FIGURE Dp-12

In the final audiogram (Figure Dp-13), the graphs for both ears show that all lines of hyperaudition have disappeared. We think now that any depressive tendency is gone for good. There have been no problems for several years, and two later audiometric checkups have shown no abnormalities.

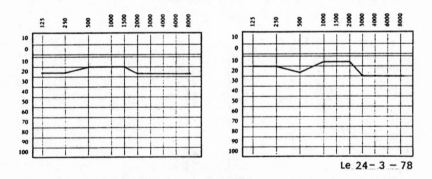

FIGURE Dp-13

The interesting factor in this case is the parallel changes in the nervous condition and the hearing abnormalities:

- improved audiogram = disappearance of depressive state

158

- setback in the audiogram = aggravation of depression
- normalization of audiogram = disappearance of problems.

ROGER

In our work with people with suicidal tendencies, this is the case that gave us the greatest concern, and I will give a more thorough account of this case than usual. My experience with this sort of case was limited at this time, and I didn't have the confidence I have acquired since then in dealing with this difficult type of situation.

In 1971 a doctor from the south of France called, asking me to see immediately a patient of his who was in the midst of a series of attacks of suicidal compulsion. The patient, a man of thirty-seven, appeared the next morning, accompanied by his wife and children. As he came through the door, he declared, "I came because Dr. X has been very devoted to me and I felt practically forced into it. But I warn you, after I leave here, I shall kill myself."

That sort of statement is difficult to put to one side, but we managed to question Roger somewhat, and found that he had mild problems of the maxillary sinus and of nasal polyps. He was a sheet metal worker, and was constantly surrounded by noise of high intensity. He had a reputation as a fighter. And for the last two years he had experienced a deep depression that had led to two suicide attempts. Medical treatment produced no result.

The ENT examination showed a slight deviation of the right nostril wall. The audiogram (Figure Dp-14) showed a bilateral and very pronounced 2-8 curve.

I explained at length and in great detail the principles of my diagnosis and treatment, and then repeated it all. I expected that the patient, clearly an intelligent man, would understand the explanation perfectly well. However, he would only answer, with a sad smile, "Thank you, Doctor, but when I leave, I'll kill myself."

Finally, in front of his wife and children, I presented him with this deal:

"I don't ask you to believe what I'm telling you, but simply to follow the treatment to the end, whatever happens, whatever unpleasant reactions you suffer. If, at the end of

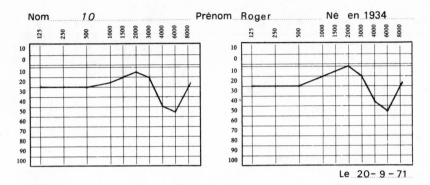

FIGURE Dp-14

the treatment, your decision remains the same, I will do nothing to keep you from it. This could be the best course for you, as it has been for others."

He replied, "Very well, Doctor, it's agreed; I shall go to the end."

The treatment began. The only reactions worth mentioning were a few pains in the left ear, insomnia which required medication, and some shaking after the ninth session.

During the sessions, Roger would sit bent over, with an empty look and say, "Only seven days left.". . . "Only six days left."

The treatment was to end on a Thursday. On Monday: "Only four days left." Tuesday: "Only three days . . ."

Tuesday was really very bad; with the fatal day approaching, there was no change in Roger's state.

Then on Wednesday, he said, "Doctor, I think you have won. This morning I asked my wife if she had not forgotten to turn the gas off before we left. It means that I am thinking of a different future than death."

The final audiogram (Figure Dp-15) showed that the 2-8 curve had disappeared. The picture was by no means all positive. The curve was still very abnormal, and could start again in the wrong direction; and the patient still appeared emotionally very vulnerable. I therefore asked him to come

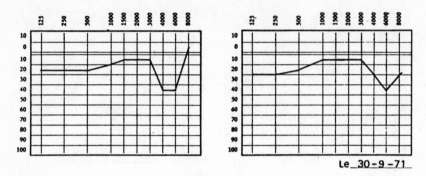

Le 30-9-71

FIGURE Dp-15

back to Annecy as soon as he noticed any symptoms of a setback.

Three months later, in a slight depressive state, Roger returned for a ten-day treatment. After four months, a routine checkup showed that his condition seemed to have stabilized at last. At that point I and my staff could admit that we had been very frightened about the course this case might follow.

Two years later I greeted in my office a smiling man, full of energy and health, looking ten years younger than he had.

It was Roger . . . bringing his wife in to be treated for depression.

AFTERWORD

by Annabel Stehli

In my book, *The Sound of a Miracle,* I tell the story of my daughter Georgiana's ordeal with autism and the role of Dr. Bérard's method of auditory training in her recovery. Bérard's book covers the technical bases, while mine covers the emotional ones, and together they document a remarkable and genuine breakthrough. The information Bérard presents is of particular value to parents of children with the disorders he addresses, primarily dyslexia and other learning disabilities, and, to some extent, autism. You have seen in the chapter on this condition that my daughter Georgie was his only complete success, although all the children he treated experienced some improvement. (He does not mention that most of the other autistic children brought to him were functioning on a far lower level than Georgie, and that the degree of their progress, although similar, was therefore not sufficient to propel them dramatically into the mainstream.)

The exciting news is that in the years since Dr. Bérard treated these children, speech pathologists, audiologists, and other professionals have been learning his technique, and auditory training has taken hold in the United States and Canada. Now there are many "Georgies," children who were once labelled autistic and who are now living normal, happy lives. As an example of this, we see many high-functioning five-year-olds with autistic features who can often be mainstreamed into first grade a few months after auditory training, particularly if they change to a school where their prior history of autism is unknown, and where normal behavior and learning ability are expected of them.

For lower-functioning children, the Giant Steps Program in Montreal is the best I have seen, and in fact is able to mainstream autistic children of Georgie's type within five years, without an aide, if they are enrolled by age 3. The parents as well as the teachers undergo months of training in the Giant Steps method, in order to provide a consistent approach around the clock.

Giant Steps, and other school systems such as Aldine in Houston and Ridgefield in New Jersey, offer auditory training as part of their program, but not all educational (and medical) professionals have been so receptive. Since my book came out and I embarked on the lecture/talk show circuit, I have encountered extensive opposition to auditory training. Twenty-five years ago I was all but burned at the stake as a refrigerator mother; now I am sometimes characterized as a charlatan, an opportunist, or a stage mother, or all three at once, as well as irresponsible for launching an untried modality with insufficient evidence, raising false hopes, and encouraging parents to spend their time and money unwisely. But now that the reports of improvement in thousands of children have gone beyond the anecdote stage, and the double-blind studies have provided encouraging data, the criticism is diminishing. Interestingly, hostility is rarely a factor when Georgie is speaking with me. Her warmth, charm, and the easygoing, relaxed state of her recovery convince even the most hardened skeptics, and her blistering indictment of the special education system which almost destroyed her is received with respectful interest.

The trouble is that auditory training seems too good to be true. Worse, if it is true, it will undermine the referral bases of many practitioners of established medicine. Some psychotherapists have greeted the effectiveness of auditory training with about as much enthusiasm as obstetricians showed for natural childbirth in the fifties. "What, women deliver their own babies?" my obstetrician said. "Ridiculous. It's safer, you say? And less painful? Better for the baby as well as the mother? Cost-effective? Nonsense." And yet within twenty years, as its excellent results became known, natural childbirth became standard procedure. In the same decade, if you wanted to call someone a fraud, you called him a chiropractor, and orthopedic surgeons were not known to refer patients to chiropractors as they frequently do now. And insurance didn't pay for it.

Dr. Bérard's work, and the consequent work of researchers like Drs. Bernard Rimland and Stephen Edelson, who have run double-blind clinical trials, make it clear that autism responds to auditory training to some degree, and learning disabilities appear to do so also. It would be better, rather than "disabilities," to refer to them as clusters of sensory processing anomalies and thereby allow some focus on the formidable assets which accompany the liabilities. When conditions are lumped together in a "disability" category, prejudice is encouraged, and a glass ceiling in special education often results.

Too many special education programs are based on the concept of managing an incurable disability, which means that the teachers may unwittingly foster underachieving in the child. Georgie, who, like most people with autism, has a phenomenally comprehensive and accurate memory, recalls every detail of her own experience in special education, and is convinced that she (in her words) "never would have made it" had she returned to her former school after auditory training. I don't wish to cast aspersions on all special education teachers, many of whom are dedicated and effective, but the teachers in Georgie's school would have expected her to perform as poorly as before, would have been looking for remaining weaknesses rather than new strengths, and would have felt threatened by the success of a new treatment strategy which they hadn't learned about in graduate school. And the threat of auditory training working so well that special education might no longer be needed was also a factor. A special ed teacher actually marched up to me at a recent conference and said, "What are you trying to do, lose me my job?"

"You, especially," I wish I'd replied, instead of standing there speechless with shock.

As things are, coping with catastrophe is what a lot of

people are paid to do, and perhaps the system's built-in bias works to ensure the maintenance of a level of catastrophe that will support the establishment that has grown up to cope with it. And the greater the disaster the greater the funding. This is not only true about the conditions discussed in this book, but about health care in this country in general. I can't imagine how it would ever be brought about, but the ancient Chinese idea of paying physicians while their patients stayed well and suspending payment when they got sick seems to make more sense than our methods, which make sickness so profitable.

I suppose that a start would be prevention, an idea that is being applied to more and more health conditions. Dr. Bérard has not discussed any causes of the sensory processing anomalies that occur in the autism, dyslexia and depression he treated, beyond a mention of ear infections, but my own and others' observations indicate that we should be exploring environmental pollution and ear infections treated repeatedly with antibiotics as the two main culprits. Dr. William Crook also argues convincingly for an important role for allergies. The poisonous nonsense, fostered in the '60s by Dr. Bruno Bettelheim, of blaming the mother for the condition has now been largely discredited, though not until after generations of families were pointlessly tortured and countless marriages destroyed— and decades of chances to examine the real causes irretrievably lost. I still hear stories of helping professionals prospecting for dysfunction and prescribing psychotherapy and drugs as the only remedies. Would they probe the psyche of the parent of a child with cerebral palsy, looking for psychogenic etiology? and yet both autism and cerebral palsy are neurological in origin.

Those of you who have read this book out of general interest in its topic will, I think, have been fascinated and moved. Parents of children with special needs will have gained conclusive evidence of a technique that can almost certainly help many children, and if motivated to investigate further, may contact the Georgiana Organization, Inc., P.O. Box 2607, Westport, CT 06880, for information. As of February, 1993, there are available across the United States and Canada 150 practitioners of the Bérard Method of auditory training.

I first heard about auditory training in 1971, when my daughter was six. On the authority of leading experts in the field at the time, I dismissed it, costing Georgie the remaining years of her already ravaged childhood. I was guilty of contempt prior to investigation, and God willing, I hope I will continue to be instrumental in sparing others the same fate.

Annabel Stehli
Westport, Connecticut

APPENDIX

SCIENTIFIC EVIDENCE FOR THE RELATIONSHIP BETWEEN HEARING AND DYSLEXIA

I hope we have amply demonstrated in this book the role of auditory problems in the process of learning speech and, subsequently, in school. This idea is not universally accepted. We have read professional articles on dyslexia and learning disabilities and have seen television programs on the same topic, in which some such statement as this was made: "We shall eliminate auditory problems from the start, except those of total deafness, because they do not belong here."

Fortunately there have been other studies refuting this absurd viewpoint, and I shall cite a few of them here.

- Document MIDY: *Collection internationale Paris-Bruxelles-Athènes-Mexico-Milan,* 1966.

  Hearing is indispensable to language formation. Therefore an accentuated auditory problem will cause linguistic difficulties and will disturb the intellectual development of the affected subject.

  The language level depends on the following conditions established by the cochlea. Heavy deafness corresponds to an absolute absence of language and expression: the child is deaf-mute. A light deafness slows down only a child with little gift for language learning. A deafness of 40 to 60 dB for conversation frequencies slows the subject down considerably, and among deaf people, only gifted individuals manage to structure, with the help of reading lips, spontaneous speech.

Auditory affliction is never an isolated problem in a child. The examination always brings forth problems in space orientation, problems in speech and articulation, as slowdown in language development. In fact, the sensorial problem appears at the language learning level and at the level of personality development.

It is at the level of language that the problems are most important. It is difficult to express sounds that one cannot control. It is the same for the adult for whom a problem of perception gives characteristic variations of the tone quality, whereas the learning and mechanism of speech were acquired a long time previously.

The reproduction of sound is hardly disturbed if well heard by a child. But if tones of some phonemes are sent out at a level not perceived, they will be poorly reproduced.

- M. Castetz, "Les retards du langage. *Concours Médical de France*, 17 April 1970.

The primary cause of slowness is deafness, and we must always keep it in mind. . . . The deaf child goes through the same steps of learning language as those who hear well, and if well stimulated, he can reach the age of 10 to 12 months without a deficiency being noticed. The hypacousic child presents an often rather difficult diagnostic problem and, if not properly identified, hypacousia (hearing deficiency) can lead to a mistaken diagnosis of behavior instability or of intellectual deficiency. At the slightest suspicion, it is necessary to have a specialized examination . . .

- *Médicographie*, April 1965. I have excerpted this brief passage from this 17-page article.

Most often, auditory problems are revealed through language problems. We can identify:
   a) the deaf who are mute for lack of sound information;
   b) the half-mute for whom vocal information is fragmented and is at the root of profound problems of pronunciation;

  c) the hard of hearing and partial deaf, who have pronunciation difficulties, in particular with Ls and Rs. . . .

• Irene and Alex Ewing.

  It is among children in school that audiometry can find systematically children who present hearing problems not too accentuated and usually undetected by the family. The advantage of this examination no longer needs to be proven. For example, it has allowed us to identify 75 children of whom 65 had pronunciation problems among 84 children who were labeled as poor students by their school.

• D. Sadek, "Demi-surdité et rééducation." *La Clinique*, 1966.

  . . . the cases of half-deafness can be misidentified in children, these being considered to be children with behavior problems or mentally retarded. . . .

• Pauget and Longraye, "Statistiques de surdité chez l'enfant." *Journal Française d'O.R.L.*, 3, 1966.

  . . . a total of about 500 children referred by their parents or instructors because of speech, concentration or school problems. . . . In 44% of the cases, it is a problem of transmission deafness. It is important not to ignore the fact, since with the proper help most of these children will catch up. Forty-seven percent of these cases of deafness stem from perception, which unfortunately does not respond well to treatment.
  . . . we notice that among children, only about one-fifth have a deficiency of more than 40 dB and a resulting serious handicap.

• Prof. Portman, "L'enfant malentendant." *Emission d'Enseignement Médico-Chirurgical*, 1969. We shall end this partial list of authors who agree that a strong parallel exists between the quality of a child's hearing and his performance in school by reproducing some sections of this article. After detailed descriptions of the speech path through the auditory circuit, the author writes:

> All breaks in this system before the age of learning, that is before the age of 2 or 3, will bring about a serious disturbance. . . . It removes all possibility of peripheral stimulation: no sound perception, therefore no creation of an internal language, hence no notion of language. This is an example of the typical deaf-mute. But it is certain that, aside from deaf-mutes, there are cases of partial deafness that are sometimes extremely unfavorable to the acquisition of language for the simple reason that the child will not always have an aptitude for language.

After a few examples of typical cases he states:

> . . . if you are faced with laziness, lack of concentration, some behavior problems, problems in language articulation, lack of language and lack of emotional behavior in the child, always think of having the young sufferer examined. He might have an auditory problem which has not been identified; and if that is so you must consult a competent otologist trained in pediatric audiology.

BIBLIOGRAPHY

The following works are mentioned to help familiarize readers with the general phenomena of hearing.

Bellier—Thèse de Doctorat. (Doctoral Thesis), Paris.

Borel-Maisonny—Langage oral et écrit (*Oral and Written Language*), Delachaux and Nestlé.

Castetz—Les retards de langage (*Delays in Language*), Concours Médical de France, April 18, 1970.

Garde—La vibration des cordes vocales et ses niveaux encéphaliques d'intégration (*Vocal Chord Vibration and Their Levels of Integration in the Brain*), Revue de Laryngologie, 1953.

Gribenski—L'audition-Que Sais-je? (*Hearing—What Do I Know?*), P.U.F. Husson—Communication à l'Académie des Sciences (*Presentation at the Academy of Sciences*), March 15 and 25, 1957.

Husson—Communication à l'Académie des Sciences (*Presentation at the Academy Sciences*), March 15 and 25, 1957.

Husson—Communication à l'Academie de Médecine (Presentation at the Academy of Medicine), June 4, 1957.

Masson—Asthme et bruit (*Asthma and Sound*), Plymouth College of Technology.

Matras—Le son-Que sais-je? (*Sound—What Do I Know?*), P.U.F.

Midy—documents, Le problème de langage (*Documents, The Problem of Language*), 1966.

Paiget and Longrate—Statistiques sur les surdités de l'enfant (*Statistics on Child Deafness*), Journal Francais d'Otorhinolaryngologie No. 3, 1966.

Portmann—L'enfant malentendant (*The Child with Poor Hearing*).

Roussey and Filippi—Direction des états psychiatriques par analyses de la voix (*The Management of Psychiatric Problems by Voice Analysis*), Tribune médicale.

Sadek—Demi-surdité et rééducation (*Partial Deafness and Retraining*), May, 1966.

Index